COPD
innovative breathing techniques

A natural, stress-free approach
to coping with chronic obstructive
pulmonary disease using the
Brice Method

Paul Brice

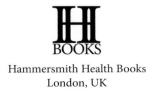

Hammersmith Health Books
London, UK

This book is dedicated to the memory of Morag Minton

First published in 2018 by Hammersmith Health Books – an imprint of
Hammersmith Books Limited
4/4A Bloomsbury Square, London WC1A 2RP, UK
www.hammersmithbooks.co.uk

British Library Cataloguing in Publication Data: A CIP record of this book is available from the
British Library.

Print ISBN 978-1-78161-122-7
Ebook ISBN 978-1-78161-123-4

Commissioning editor: Georgina Bentliff
Designed and typeset by: Julie Bennett of Bespoke Publishing Ltd
Cover design by: Julie Bennett of Bespoke Publishing Ltd
Index: Dr Laurence Errington
Production: Helen Whitehorn of Path Projects Ltd
Printed and bound by: TJ International Ltd, Padstow, Cornwall
Cover photo: Antonio Guillem, Shutterstock

Contents

Important safety advice for the reader

Before following any of the advice contained in this book, it is recommended that you consult with your doctor if you are in doubt as to the suitability of the exercises.

If, like many people who suffer from COPD, you are very inactive, read the section on 'Monitoring any pain' in the Introduction (page 9). This specifically advises you on what you should be able to do and what you should avoid.

Foreword

Presumably the reason you are reading this book is because you or a loved one is experiencing problems with breathing. Getting out of breath is not always pleasant; however, it is normal. It is a natural response when your body needs more oxygen and energy when you do something that requires physical effort. Getting out of breath when we exert ourselves is a positive reaction and is usually viewed as a normal response to increased activity.

However, some people get out of breath every day when they're not physically exerting themselves. They unexpectedly find it difficult or uncomfortable to breathe, and may feel they can't control their breathing. This long-term breathlessness is known as 'chronic breathlessness'. It often develops gradually and lasts for weeks, months or years. Sometimes people also cough, bring up phlegm or feel wheezy (British Lung Foundation 2018).

Breathlessness is not only a physical symptom. It can also affect how we feel about things. An episode of breathlessness which has made us feel frightened or anxious will affect how we cope with the same situation when we next encounter it. This can lead to avoiding certain situations and allowing the fear of breathlessness to stop us living our lives as completely as we would wish.

Over the past 30 years working with people with breathing problems, I have been exposed to many methods of trying to counteract the symptoms of lung diseases, particularly chronic obstructive lung (or 'pulmonary') disease (COPD). General practitioners and specialists can refer suitable people with breathing problems to local services providing pulmonary rehabilitation programmes.

Over the past 15 years I have managed the local pulmonary rehabilitation service and have firsthand experience of how these programmes can enhance the lives of people with lung diseases. These invaluable programmes are particularly beneficial for people with COPD. Anyone with this condition should ask for a referral as they can dramatically improve how they cope with their breathlessness.

The Brice Method has developed from Paul Brice working with colleagues in the NHS over many years. Paul is an inspirational leader in the area of breathlessness management. His insight into the individual's fears regarding their challenging breathing is instinctive and within one session he can reduce fear and reinstate hope in the lives of people who have been severely affected both physically and mentally by their breathlessness.

I have worked closely with Paul over the past nine years and have always been impressed by his results. I have confidence in his abilities to look at innovative ways of helping individuals cope better with a condition which cannot be cured. Just because a condition cannot be cured does not mean that it cannot be helped.

I would encourage anyone with lung disease to read this book and to lend it to their Respiratory Health Care Professional to inspire others to adopt the safe and effective Brice Method for helping to manage breathlessness.

Heather Matthews RN RM BSC (HON) MSC
Independent Respiratory Nurse Specialist
UK

About the author

Paul Brice is a Sports Scientist and Clinical Exercise Specialist and has been working in the field of Exercise Rehabilitation for more than 20 years. A former international athlete, with a Joint Honours BSc in Sports Science and Biology, Paul has worked in the health and fitness sectors since 1987. Paul worked as a physical activity lead for the Great Yarmouth and Waveney PCT for seven years, working on promoting physical activity to improve health.

With business partner Spencer McCormack, Paul helped set up the first commercial health club to be based within an NHS Hospital in the UK and has worked for the NHS on a number of pilot schemes using physical activity in conjunction with conventional NHS treatment to help improve health outcomes.

Since 2009 Paul has been working alongside the award-winning Respiratory Nursing Team, at the James Paget University Hospital, Great Yarmouth. (They won the Association of Respiratory Nurses, Nursing Team of the Year 2016.) Paul is one of the innovators of the BEET (Breathing, Exercise, Education, Training) programme. BEET is a community gym-based pulmonary rehabilitation programme that has had over 2500 patients referred to it over the last nine years.

Paul has a strong belief that sensible movement and moderate physical activity are two of the key foundations of a healthy, balanced body and mind. He works with patients by explaining the impact inactivity and immobility can have on the many health systems in the body, to help them understand that they may be able to reverse their health issues if they put a little effort into being more active and more mobile. Paul shows patients what they should aim for and how they can progress, and helps to keep them motivated to reach their goals. These beliefs and approach have been fundamental to the development of the Brice Method.

Paul is passionate about making a difference and now works delivering exercise rehabilitation programmes and personal training for private clients, under his business Brice Exercise Specialists Ltd.

Acknowledgements

Firstly, I would like to thank my oldest and best friend, Don Thompson. He would not realise how influential his musings have been since we started working together in the same company, on the same day, over 30 years ago. Don has been a consistent fount of knowledge, and the worn-out books and suggested reading list he gave me over 20 years ago when he was studying osteopathy, Rolfing, Hellerwork and other body working techniques, prompted me to look outside the conventional sport and fitness box.

I need to acknowledge Heather Matthews, Carol Nicholls, Fiona Lang, Lesley Barber and Maria Hunter from the Respiratory Nursing Team at the James Paget University Hospital. Heather, Carol and Fiona have all been instrumental in enabling me to develop my method. They have played vital roles in the development of BEET, the innovative community pulmonary rehabilitation programme. Their drive and determination to meet patients' needs are why they were recognised as the ARNS, UK Respiratory Nursing Team of the Year in 2016.

Finally, I would probably never have got around to finding a publisher for this book if it had not been for one of my former patients, Morag Minton. Morag had very severe COPD and was told her best opportunity to live a full life was a double lung transplant. She was referred to me having just spent eight weeks in hospital with a very severe chest infection over the Christmas and New Year. When I met her, Morag was very down, as weak as a kitten, and her shoulders were so tight we could hardly prise them from her ears. She spent most of her day hunched up trying to recover from the previous breath she had just taken. She had been a top fitness presenter and loved rock climbing. She took on board the exercises I gave her, and her breathing started improving almost immediately. She did her daily exercises until she could attend the gym, where she ended up not only getting stronger herself, but also talking to novice patients when they looked a little lost.

Morag continually pestered me to write this book. She had done exhaustive research, and nothing had worked for her until she did the exercises that were shown to her. She was insistent that it was important that other people with COPD got the chance to try them.

Amazingly, within seven months Morag was strong enough to have her lung transplant. I had planned for her to work for me after her operation, to train as an exercise specialist. Unfortunately, whilst her lungs transplanted well and initially worked, a complication from the operation meant that she did not survive.

As I complete my final draft, I wish to dedicate this book to the memory of Morag Minton.

Illustrations: I took all the photographs myself and the bar charts were devised by me and refined by Hammersmith Books. The following are included with permission from Shutterstock: Figure 1.1 Tewan Banditrukkanka; Figure 1.3 Alila Medical Media. Figure 1.5 Adapted from: Alison McConnell, *Respiratory Muscle Training; Theory and Practice*, Elsevier, Oxford, 2013. Other illustrations by Tech-Set Ltd, Gateshead.

Introduction

What is COPD?

COPD (chronic obstructive pulmonary disease) is an umbrella term used to classify a number of conditions of the lungs that impair breathing. Bronchitis and emphysema are the two most frequent conditions under this umbrella term, but there is a whole range of complaints and illnesses that are labelled under the same banner. The meanings of the terms which make up the acronym are as follows:

chronic: it is a long-term condition and does not go away
obstructive: your airways are narrowed, so it's harder to breathe
pulmonary: it affects your lungs
disease: it is a medical condition.

The UK's Health and Social Care Information Centre questioned medical practices in England and reported in March 2015 that over 1,034,578 people were registered with their GPs as having a diagnosis of COPD, an increase of over 2% in a single year.

Many other people with breathing difficulties go undiagnosed and/or do not go to their GP for help or diagnosis. This means the issue may be even more common than these statistics indicate. This is borne out by The Health Survey for England 2010, which estimated that 6% of adults had probable airflow limitations consistent with COPD. If this 6% figure were true it would be equivalent to around 3 million people in the UK.

This book is the culmination of thousands of hours of work with a wide range of breathing and lung conditions under the banner of COPD. It includes a section that details the personal feedback from hundreds of patients suffering from COPD, and is designed to help readers understand how their breathing can be adversely affected by the way they behave, stand, sit and move, but conversely how they might be able to improve their breathing by doing these simple everyday activities differently.

The results from those who complete the programme are quite staggering. I have found that patients' blood oxygen saturation increased during the first session with me from an average of 94.5% to an average of 97.6%. Blood oxygen saturation gives an immediate indication of how much oxygen is being absorbed into the bloodstream from the lungs, and is used extensively to monitor patients' progress. I have also found that patients report on average a 64.5% improvement in their quality of breath within the first session. Hopefully, using the techniques in this book you will benefit as much as one of my average patients. You will get the opportunity to try this out for yourself if you do the first Landmark test at the end of this Introduction (page 13), and then re-do this test as recommended at various stages in the book.

The development of the Brice Method has, in part, been driven by the desire to find an alternative early stage intervention that might be able to delay the need for expensive pharmacological treatment of COPD. The development of the programme has been gradual. Many of the exercises are treatments that may have been used by previous generations of medical practitioners and, in some respects, it uses skills that may have been overlooked when 'high tech' alternatives were developed. As with most other lifestyle-related conditions, the use of physical activity for COPD is aimed at the causes of the condition, not the symptoms.

Built into this book is a series of simple exercises to help a person with COPD listen to their body, understand their dysfunctional breathing patterns and learn to manage and cope with their condition.

Whilst there can be no guarantee that the Brice Method will definitely help every person with COPD, the vast majority of patients have found this innovative programme useful to some degree or another. Most of the patients who have gone through it have said that the programme has dramatically improved their lives.

The method is designed to be simple to implement. It is based upon the idea that we should use our lungs the way nature intended. Despite the method being simple, patients who have done the programme have reported that there are profound changes that have helped them breathe better, move better and live better.

Who is the book written for?

This book is aimed specifically at the layperson with COPD, and as such you will not find numbered references or reading lists, as it would affect the flow of what is essentially a self-help book.

If you have COPD you will probably have been given an idea of how badly you are affected by your condition. All COPD patients are given a number from 1 to 5 as to how much of an impact their breathlessness has on their daily living. This is called the 'MRC grading'. The five divisions are listed and explained in the box.

Medical Research Council Breathlessness Scale
MRC1:   Not troubled by breathlessness except on strenuous exertion
MRC2:   Short of breath when hurrying, or walking up a slight hill
MRC3:   Walks more slowly than other people, stops after a mile or so, or stops after walking for 15 minutes at own pace
MRC4:   Stops for breath after walking for about 100 yards, or after a few minutes on level ground
MRC5:   Too breathless to leave the house, or breathless when undressing.

As the Brice Method is a very low-key programme of advice and exercise, it is suited to all five levels of MRC grading. The programme aims to assist those with mild breathlessness to learn what they can do themselves to help prevent their breathlessness worsening due to poor lifestyle choices. Conventional pulmonary rehabilitation has previously been deemed unsuitable for those COPD patients with an MRC5 grading. This is due to the nature of the physical exercises in that programme being too intensive for people who are severely affected by their breathlessness. Unlike conventional programmes, the Brice Method has been shown to work effectively with MRC5 patients. This is partly due to its graded, step-by-step approach, focusing on low-level tasks before it moves on gradually to more active stages. The very breathless patients can start off with hardly any exertion at all, only progressing when they have mastered the stage they are working on. If they find that they are unable to progress beyond a certain stage due to other health conditions, then they will still have benefited up to that point.

Why the book was written

I feel that the Brice Method has come about as I have a different perspective on breathing from many of my counterparts. I believe that my background as a competitive athlete helped me to develop a critical eye on how the body can limit a person's ability to breathe, and ultimately limit their physical performance.

During my athletic career, I was always aware that I had a habit of sizing up my opponents before a competition. Being a multi-event athlete, I regularly competed against shot putters, long jumpers, sprinters, hurdlers, pole-vaulters, javelin throwers and long-distance runners. By sizing them up, I don't just mean the opponent's height and weight or bulk; I mean that I looked at their posture and their movement patterns. Nearly every athletic event has a breathing pattern that goes with it. The oomph you need for a shot putt contrasts with the rhythm of the hurdles, and the strong control needed for the pole vault contrasted with the relaxed requirement of longer distance running events.

As an athlete I was lucky enough to be on the first wave of guinea pigs in the UK who routinely had their physiological capacities tested. These tests included measurements of the power output and strength of our muscles, our flexibility, as well as a plethora of other tests. One of the tests was the lung function test, which is the same test dreaded by most COPD patients. Being competitive, I quickly learned how to try to beat the tests to maximise my score. It was natural for me to try and open my lungs up as fully as possible to get the best score, something that has influenced my working with my patients.

When I started working with people with COPD I immediately wanted to use my experience and knowledge to help them be more active, especially when so many of them looked like they had forgotten how their lungs worked. It is probably not surprising that the techniques I used to get the extra 10% out of my lungs as an athlete would provide an even greater benefit for people with lung and breathing problems.

Pharmacological treatment of COPD

Over the last two decades, the advances in medical knowledge and respiratory medicine have been extraordinary. The research and understanding of the scientific minutiae of the potential causes and intricate treatment of specific issues of impaired breathing have undoubtedly helped many millions of people.

Whilst it is wonderful that we have these powerful tools, many practitioners are now starting to ask if we are using these drugs too readily. In the UK, and in other advanced countries, we are starting to see drug resistance. It may be that we have become a little too quick to use these highly advanced treatments to manage symptoms of breathlessness, especially at the early stages of diseases such as COPD, where patients should possibly have the chance to address the lifestyle issues that may have caused the symptoms in the first place.

When I treat people who have had COPD for many years, and are showing the obvious effects of long-term steroid and antibiotic use, and I show them the simple exercises that start the Brice Method journey, some of the more knowledgeable even ask me, 'Why haven't I been shown this before?' In my clinic I have had up to 98% of my COPD patients say they have felt significant benefit to their breathing from a more holistic approach to their initial treatment using the Brice Method. It may be that the cost of doing clinical trials to demonstrate the effectiveness of interventions is prohibitive for simple interventions like this. In the 'real world', it is usually only pharmaceuticals that can reap the financial return to justify such monetary investment.

Holistic approach

The Brice Method aims to look holistically at the individual patient, and what might be contributing to their breathlessness, bearing in mind other conditions, not just the lungs.

Many COPD patients have specific illnesses, or conditions, directly linked to their breathlessness. Others have medical issues that would appear at first glance to have little or no association with their breathing problems. How could a patient with arthritis and two knee replacements have those two issues associated with their breathlessness? Or, how could a patient with chronic back pain that has debilitated them for a decade have been predisposed to present at a COPD clinic? The answer is quite simple, but often overlooked.

In reality, many of the patients that present at clinic have either one significant, or a number of, health or lifestyle issues that may in some way have led them to be more inactive. Some of these issues are physical, like a leg or back problem; others can be psychological. A large number of the elderly patients are clearly resigned to having poor health because they have been told by well-meaning people that 'there is nothing more than can be done, it is the effect of aging'.

True breathlessness often creeps up on you

To explain how easy it is for breathing problems to creep up on you, health professionals use a diagram called the 'spiral of de-conditioning' (see Figure 1) to demonstrate the typical onset of breathing problems in patients with COPD. The 'spiral' is commonly used in pulmonary rehabilitation programmes to explain how a patient can become less and less able over time due to relative inactivity.

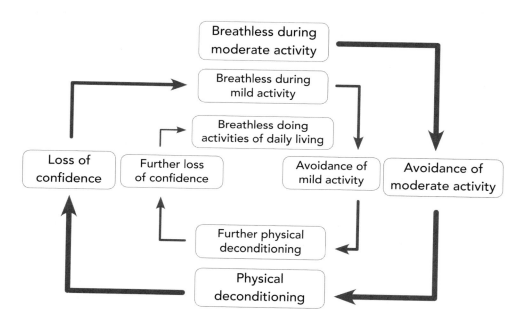

Figure 1: *The spiral of deconditioning/breathlessness*

This spiral of ever-reducing ability can take a considerable period of time to manifest itself. Its gradual creeping effect means that some people will only realise that they have been getting worse when they really can't do something simple like stand up from a chair. Other people will find this process can be extremely rapid. For example, a long stay in hospital or a severe chest infection can mean you go from being able to do relatively moderate activities to not going out at all within a week or two.

Deconditioning like this over time is effectively a Catch-22 situation. The negative spiral continues until, eventually, even the slightest physical movement becomes challenging, and it is at this stage patients will present at one of my COPD clinics, saying that they find any exercise makes them feel stressed or panicky.

The good news is, for most people, the cycle is reversible to some degree or other. Whilst I can never promise that people will regain their confidence and physical capacities in full, with consistent and gradually progressing activities, nearly all COPD patients I work with feel they have managed to regain some control of what was a downward slide to complete loss of independence.

How to use this book

This book has been structured in four stages, which mimic the way in which I would teach a client in my clinic.

- First, I explain in detail about where the lungs are and how they should work. This means you may get an insight into why you will be doing the later exercises.
- Secondly, I cover some of the main breathing issues people with COPD tend to demonstrate.
- Thirdly, I explain why you should adapt your posture to breathe better before I even start to give you any physical exercises.

The exercise component of the Brice Method (stage 4) only begins at Chapter 5. It starts with upper body exercises, moves on to lower body exercises, then covers breathing on the move and finally how to develop more oomph.

The book then covers further information about living with breathlessness.

You will be expected to do regular daily homework exercises to help you undo some of the bad habits that you will undoubtedly have developed over the years. To help you locate these exercises easily, they are shaded dark grey on the outer edge of the page, with the name of the relevant exercise written on them.

Your attention will be drawn to three key 'landmarks' throughout the book where you can assess the quality of your breathing before and during the programme. These landmarks mirror the measures that I use with my clinical patients. I have found that using these 'self-test' measures has given focus, confidence and adherence to up to 95% of these patients.

The first of the three landmarks is undertaken before you even start Chapter 1, and provides you with the reference point to measure your full progress against. I have provided the results of 302 COPD patients in Addendum 1 (page 135), so that you can compare your results with those of my clinical patients.

There are some exercises that will benefit from some equipment. I have explained in Addendum 2 (page 141) how you can start off without investing any real money, and what options you have if you need to buy some more suitable equipment once you have full confidence in the programme.

If you have other medical conditions that are equally limiting to you as your breathlessness, or even more so, you should re-read the initial warning advice right at the start of the book and consult your GP before starting the programme, as well as following the advice on monitoring pain and discomfort that comes next in this Introduction.

Monitoring any pain

If you have recently been advised by your doctor to exercise, or you are starting out on this programme from scratch, the likelihood is that you will have done very little, or no real, physical activity for some time. As I have said, chronic conditions like COPD creep up on you slowly and you may not realise how rusty and 'graunchy' your once healthy, active body has become until you start to move it outside of your usual limited range of motion.

Discomfort or pain

Jane Fonda, one of the first high-profile fitness leaders in the 1970s, had a mantra of 'no pain, no gain'. Some people still have this mantra in mind when they think about exercising, and the prospect of having to exercise hard could be one of the reasons that they have avoided exercise at all costs. Fortunately, our understanding of exercise, or better still physical activity, has moved on immensely in the last 40 years and I would hazard a guess that even Fonda herself might advise against her formerly gung-ho approach after having had two hip replacements. If you had any worries that the Brice Method was going to ask you to work hard, rest assured, this is not the case.

However, to say that you can go through the entire programme feeling absolutely no discomfort or pain would be a lie. One of the aims is to help you develop and adapt to a new, more active lifestyle, but the main objective of the Brice Method is to teach you to move without feeling out of control, especially not becoming uncomfortably breathless.

Pain is something that should be considered useful when it comes to physical activity. Our nervous system is designed to quickly tell us when things are not right, and, at its simplest, has helped humankind to develop to where we are today by avoiding threats to our survival. When it comes to exercise, pain is a great measure of what should be done and what should not be done.

Most of my patients have been relatively sedentary for some time, not moving their limbs or their bodies very much. Usually they have been so inactive that some of the simple movements in the first set of exercises designed to mobilise the upper body may initiate pain in the chest, neck or shoulders.

You will need to realise that pain is relative. Some people have higher pain thresholds than others. It has been found that people with breathing disorders who have low levels of oxygen in their bloodstream are more susceptible to chronic pain, but can also have a heightened sensitivity to pain. The good news is that many of the hyper-sensitive patients I work with find that their pain awareness reduces with gentle, sensible physical activity.

Pain guidance

Rather than simply giving up or totally avoiding the exercises, I have some guidance as follows.

- Try a movement and if 'pain' arises, stop the movement and return to the starting position of the exercise.
- If the pain is dull and achy, and if it dissipates and goes away quickly, then this feeling is not pain but is really discomfort.
- Check your body alignment against the exercise advice given and repeat; usually this will make things feel easier. If not, don't worry, time and repetition will help.
- By repeating the movement, the joints, ligaments, tendons, fascia and muscles all warm up and start to mobilise, and the range of motion generally increases.

The above sensations are either 'discomfort' or 'good pain', and once your body has overcome the shock that you are asking it to move, you will soon be reassured that it is acceptable, even normal, to feel something like this.

Caution
- If a movement causes a severe, sharp, stabbing pain then this is not such a good sign, and is an indication of 'bad pain'.
- If the pain does not subside within 30 seconds, then that is also a sign that it is 'bad pain' that should be avoided until you are sure you aren't doing something incorrectly.

If you do get sharp, severe pain with a movement, even if the pain is very severe, it does not necessarily mean that you are a lost cause, and you should give up. Before you discount an exercise, you must ensure that you are not holding your body in an incorrect posture before you start. For example, it is common for someone who has not used their arms for a while to be hunched over, and their shoulders to be stuck in a rut. By squeezing your shoulder blades backwards and together behind your back, you can usually enable your arms to move more freely and naturally.

Warning
If you have tried the above and want further guidance, you should either seek further advice from a qualified fitness specialist or see your doctor. You will have to be the judge as to when you may need external help, as only you can know how your body feels.

In the end, it will be up to you to create your own pain monitoring language. Gradually you can then use this to measure how much pain or discomfort is right for you, as well as checking that it is getting easier and less painful and not the other way around. This pain language will be your long-term guide as to how hard and for how long you can happily be physically active in the future.

Not everyone will be capable of progressing through the full programme. Some of you may have very severe bodily or health restrictions, and you will have to decide when you should stop. You need only progress to where your body realistically allows.

Keeping track of your progress

There are two ways that you can monitor and track your progress through the Brice Method.

Landmark self-tests

The first measure is the Landmark self-tests that I have mentioned before and that you should do at three specific times throughout the book. The idea here is that you will be able to assess your awareness of your breath, and how you feel you are breathing at these three key stages. The first landmark test follows this Introduction. It will then be repeated after Chapter 4 (page 56) and after Chapter 7 (page 91).

Daily exercise record sheet

The second measure of your progress will help you track the daily homework exercises that you will be given along the way. You can decide which exercises you wish to do at each stage, and wish to carry on with throughout the programme, and you can use the daily exercise record sheet on page 12, to track each week's activities. This is a very simple tracking sheet to use for your practice on the exercise stages of the programme, where you have to practise regularly to develop a new healthy habit.

You will find record sheets covering a five-week period in Addendum 2 (page 145) for ease of photocopying, or you can download a copy of the record sheets from my website, www.paulbrice.net.

Now it is time to do your first Landmark self-test.

	Monday	Tuesday	Wednesday	Thursday	Friday	Saturday	Sunday
Early morning							
Mid morning							
Afternoon							
Evening							

Table 1: *Practice record sheet – mark an 'X' in the relevant box for each time you do one group of the exercise routines.*

Landmark 1

Important: Before you go any further, to get the most benefit from this book you should ensure you try the following self-test exercise first.

It will act as a reference point for you to measure your progress, and you will be asked to repeat it twice more through the book.

Self-test 1

Take a deep breath, and think about where you can feel the air inside your body. Draw on the picture of the torso below where you feel the air going in your body.

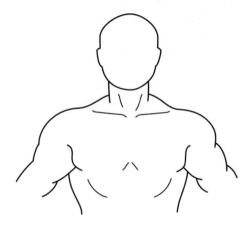

Once you have drawn the full extent of where you feel the air go into your chest, I would like you to note down how you would rate the quality of this breath on a scale of 1 to 10.

1	2	3	4	5	6	7	8	9	10
Poor				Average			Good		Fantastic

Note down your score so you can compare this with the two further self-tests you will do later in the book.

Chapter 1

Knowing your body

> ◊ **Know where your lungs are**
> ◊ **Lung structure**
> ◊ **How the lungs work**
> ◊ **Healthy lungs compared with COPD lungs**
> ◊ **The muscles involved in breathing**
> ◊ **The oxygen demand of breathing**
> ◊ **The control of breathing**

The vast majority of people go throughout life without ever having to consider their breathing. For some, the first time they pay any attention to their lungs is when they get close to their last breath. As I work almost daily with people with COPD, I find that breathing can preoccupy their minds for considerable periods of the day. What amazes me is how little most of these COPD patients know about the workings of their lungs, so I always take time to explain the basic structure and function of the respiratory system so that they get a gist of what I will be asking them to aim towards throughout the Brice Method. There are certain structures of the body that play pivotal roles in healthy breathing, and others that can contribute to breathlessness. You will need to be able to identify these structures as you go through this book, and you will eventually be able to feel yourself using parts of your body in a way that will help, not hinder, your breathing.

Not all the COPD patients I see are completely oblivious to how they can control their breathing. Many people will have learnt particular breathing techniques through activities they have done throughout their lives. Some people will have sung, or played a wind instrument, and learned how to control their breath to make music. Others may have played a sport where the manner of breathing is pivotal to performance, and others may have had a job where activities have required them to breathe in a certain way. I find this reference point can be very useful; if you can cast your mind back to an activity in your life where you have had to control your breathing to some degree, this may help you take on board the information in this book more readily. If you have never done anything where you have had to think about your breathing, don't worry. This book is designed to take you through each stage of the process. One of my ex-patients, who was in his late nineties, put into words what I was thinking when he learned to breathe in a stress-free way: 'You have taught an old dog a new trick!'

Important reminder
If you decide not to do Landmark 1 (self-test, page 13) prior to reading on, you are highly unlikely to recognise what improvements you are making as you progress through the programme. If you are serious about learning how to breathe more effectively, you will need to do the self-test and record the outcomes, so you can refer back to it at a later date.

I have found that the first thing you need to do to help you improve your breathing is to understand where your lungs are, and how they are designed to work. It is my experience that it is only when you know this information that you can fully understand where you could be going wrong and what you can do to improve your breathing.

Know where your lungs are

Strange though it may seem, the vast majority of patients that I see have absolutely no idea of where their lungs are located, and have almost no concept of their size and capacity. Once I have asked patients about their medical history and their breathing has settled down, I ask them to take a deep breath and tell me where their lungs are positioned. Most simply gesture to the general area of the chest, looking at me as if I am a bit daft bothering to ask them such an obvious question. It is a couple of seconds later when they struggle to explain exactly where their lungs are, that they realise that, even though they have a lung condition, they know very little about the organ that limits their lives so dramatically.

At this point, I take the opportunity to show my patients a picture of a normal set of lungs (see Figure 1.1). When patients see that their lungs take up almost the entirety of the inside of the rib cage, some start to get an inkling of where their problems might lie, especially if they can feel the air going only a little way into the chest in the self-test exercise, Landmark 1. (Hopefully you will have done this exercise, recorded your 1–10 score, and written down a short description of how the breath felt to you. Sorry to keep on about this, but it really is important.)

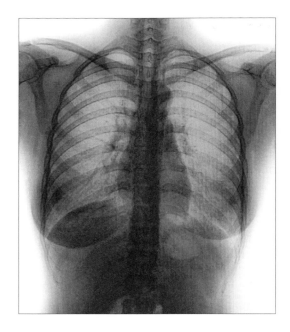

Figure 1.1: *Normal healthy lungs – the lungs almost entirely fill the rib cage*

Lung structure

The next step I take is to teach a patient how the lungs are structured, and how this structure affects their proper functioning. I will quickly run through this using a diagram of the anatomy of the respiratory system (see Figure 1.2). The area occupied by the lungs is known as the thorax, and the parts of the spine associated with this area (the thoracic spine) are called the thoracic vertebrae.

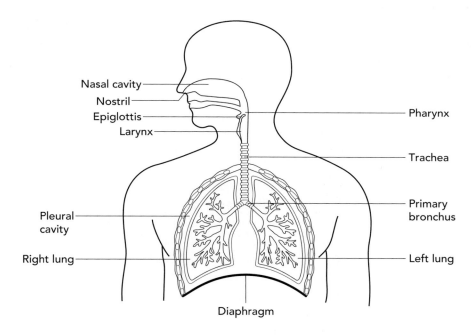

Figure 1.2: *Anatomy of the respiratory system*

Looking at Figures 1.1 and 1.2, probably the first thing you will notice is how enormous the lungs actually are. I find it useful to compare the lungs to sponges that almost completely fill the inside of the rib cage. Also inside the rib cage there is a gap for the heart, plus the tube that leads to the gut (the oesophagus), and a few blood vessels and nerve bundles (not shown here). The rib cage is designed to protect the fragile lungs, but to do so whilst still allowing the chest to be mobile enough for the lungs to work effectively. This structure is also flexible enough to assist with relatively complex body movements like walking, throwing, lifting and carrying, not to mention maintaining an upright stance.

You are already likely to know that the primary role of the lungs is to draw air into the body, extract the oxygen from the air, and make it available to the bloodstream to circulate round the body. The lungs also help get rid of carbon dioxide as well as heat, both of which are waste products of the body, as it uses up the oxygen. Oxygen is essential to help power every living cell in your body, transforming glucose into energy. Every cell requires oxygen to function effectively, and this is why the respiratory system is so important – ultimately it is key to our survival.

I feel it is vital to emphasise that the overall capacity of the lungs is ultimately linked to the expansion and contraction of the rib cage and the cavity that houses the lungs. This will be explored many times throughout this book. The lungs sit above the abdominal mass of the liver, stomach, gut and other organs. They are physically separated from the abdominal mass by an extremely strong dome-like muscle called the diaphragm.

Inhalation (breathing in) causes air to be drawn in through the nose via the nasal cavity, or directly in through the mouth. This air passes the pharynx inside the head, and then into the larynx, and down the windpipe. The windpipe, or 'trachea', is a thick cartilage-ringed pipe that takes the air down the neck into the main structure of the lungs. The trachea splits into two primary bronchi that allow air into the left and right lungs. These in turn split into ever-smaller pipes until the air reaches the minute bronchioles. Oxygen does not transfer into the bloodstream directly from these pipes; they merely transport the air into the active part of the lungs. The active part, where the oxygen is absorbed into the bloodstream, is made up of structures called 'alveoli'.

All of these structures are shown in Figure 1.3.

There are literally millions of alveoli in an adult lung, and they have the ability to expand and contract rather like a sponge. If you were to take a healthy lung from a small adult, and spread out all the alveoli on the floor, the surface area would take up the size of a badminton court. Do the same for a large adult, and the surface area would be closer to the size of a tennis court. Once you understand that such large surface areas are involved in transferring oxygen into the bloodstream, is it little wonder that the human body can do extraordinary feats of physical activity?

For the less healthy lung, smoking, pollution, disease or illness may have had the

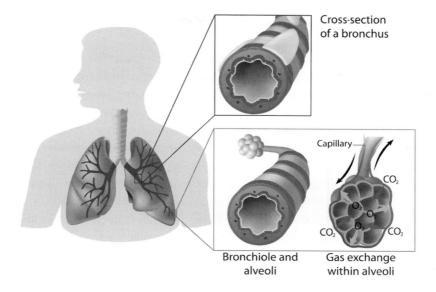

Cross-section of a bronchus

Capillary

CO_2

O_2 O_2

CO_2 O_2 CO_2

Bronchiole and alveoli

Gas exchange within alveoli

Figure 1.3: *Bronchi, bronchial tree and alveoli*

effect of damaging some areas of the alveoli, even affecting the elasticity of some of the smaller tubes that feed the alveoli. These damaged areas reduce the amount of space that is useable for the transfer of oxygen from the lungs into the bloodstream. The good news is that whilst areas of the lung may have been damaged, the remaining space is usually large enough to allow for day-to-day activities in all but the most severe cases of COPD.

I find it is reassuring to tell my patients that whilst their badminton court- or tennis court-sized space may be damaged because of their illness, they are likely to still have plenty of lung remaining. Visualising the tennis court, they are probably still going to be able to play on the smaller singles court, rather than the full doubles court. Whilst adventurous humans may need the badminton/tennis court-sized surface area of lungs to do extreme activities, like climbing Mount Everest or winning the Tour de France cycle race, much less 'floor space' is required to climb a flight of stairs or take the train to Paris. Most COPD patients have much simpler objectives.

How the lungs work – the pressure gradient

The air we breathe is a gas, and gases have properties that enable them to be moved simply from one area to another without using up very much energy. Gases move from areas of high pressure to areas of relative low pressure, and the speed at which the flow takes place depends, in the main, on the variation between the two pressures. Think about how the expansion of the chest cavity would cause the air pressure in the lungs to drop, and once the pressure is lower than the outside air, the gas will be sucked in automatically.

A COPD patient's lungs are usually as sensitive to small variations in air pressure as a barometer. Many COPD patients have yet to realise that their breathing becomes laboured when the external air pressure is low. This can help explain to some extent why on some days you can breathe more easily and on others you may not. Just as hill walkers will notice the reduction in the air pressure as they ascend a mountain, COPD patients will struggle when the air pressure is low.

It is important to understand that the structure of a healthy lung is extremely spongy and malleable. It is this sponginess that enables lung tissue to expand and contract with the chest cavity, drawing air in, and also helping push the air out with relatively little effort. Until you developed COPD it is likely that you rarely thought about the fact you were taking approximately 15 breaths a minute, every minute of every day. As it makes sense that anything which prevents the lungs from expanding or contracting will ultimately restrict a person's ability to breathe, I feel it should be the first thing to be looked at before other forms of treatment or medication are recommended.

Healthy lungs compared with COPD lungs

Normal, gentle breathing does not use the full capacity of the lungs, as the lungs have a considerable reserve volume that can be accessed when the body needs additional oxygen. This is even the case for most COPD patients. The approximate capacity of a healthy male lung is compared with that of a typical COPD lung in Figure 1.4. The normal breath we take in at rest, or during very slight movement, is called the **tidal volume**. This provides enough oxygen for the body's basic functions and is shown in grey on the diagram. The tidal volume of a healthy lung may be 500 ml, whereas in the COPD lung it may only be 300 ml. Each lung also has to have a certain amount

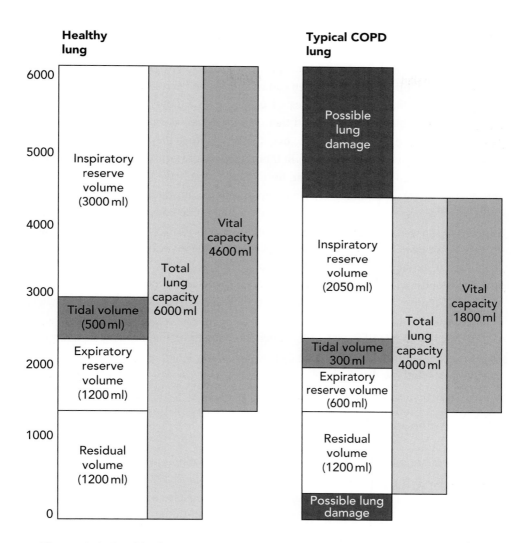

Figure 1.4: *Healthy lungs compared with COPD lungs (approximate capacities)*

of air in it to prevent it from collapsing in on itself, and this is shown as the **residual volume**, which is approximately 1200 ml. The **vital capacity** is the actual amount of air the lungs can use before they collapse on themselves. In a healthy lung, you will see that the vital capacity is approximately 4600 ml. If you compare that with the COPD lung at approximately 1800 ml, you will notice the possible area of lung damage massively limits the overall ability of the COPD lung.

As I mentioned previously in this chapter, the air has to be drawn deep into the lungs to reach the alveoli before the oxygen can be transported across into the bloodstream. The alveoli are like minute bunches of grapes with a network of capillaries (the smallest type of blood vessel) round them. Once the air is in the alveoli, oxygen is drawn from it into the bloodstream, eventually reaching the red blood cells. If the red blood cells have enough oxygen in them, the transfer of oxygen into the blood is generally limited. If there is a demand for oxygen in the body, the oxygen is absorbed into the bloodstream immediately, and carbon dioxide, produced as a waste material, travels in the opposite direction into the alveoli simultaneously. Because oxygen is capable of diffusing across only the cell membranes of the alveoli, you not only need to get the air deep enough into your lungs to reach the alveoli, but you also have to keep the air in the air sacs of the alveoli long enough for the oxygen to be absorbed into the bloodstream. Unfortunately, most COPD patients I meet tend to take quick, short and shallow breaths, especially when they are active, and this will ultimately limit their ability to exercise.

The fast breath rate of most COPD patients is something that needs to be addressed before quiet comfortable breathing can be achieved, again something that will be explored in detail later in the book.

The muscles involved in breathing

Whilst there are numerous muscles that influence breathing to some degree, I find it is best to teach my patients that there are three primary muscle groups involved in breathing. Figure 1.5 shows the location of the main muscles of breathing, along with other, secondary, muscle groups, that assist with breathing to some degree. You can refer back to this diagram as you read on.

The diaphragm

The muscle with the most profound effect on normal breathing is the diaphragm. It is a large, dome-shaped muscle that attaches to the lower ribs, separating the lungs and chest cavity from the abdominal cavity. During inhalation, the diaphragm actively contracts downwards to draw air into the expanding lungs. It relaxes automatically,

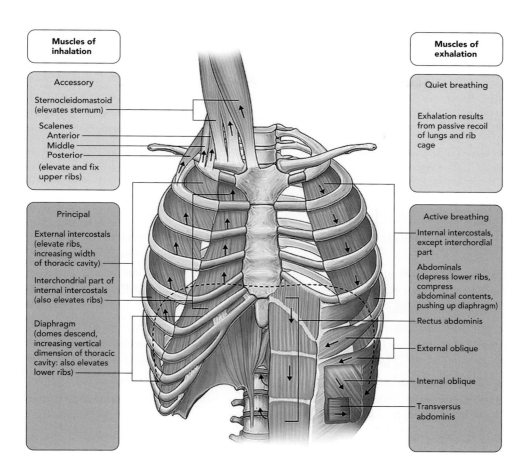

Figure 1.5 *The muscles involved in breathing*

aiding the lungs to recoil during exhalation (breathing out). When it is working effectively, the diaphragm can be responsible for as much as 80% of air flow. It is, however, easily restricted in its efforts as it relies on both the position of the ribcage to allow it to work effectively, and the muscles surrounding the abdomen to pressurise the abdominal mass for it to work against.

Muscles between the ribs

The next most effective group of muscles involved in breathing are the intercostals. There are two sets of intercostal muscles and they each attach between the individual ribs: the internal and the external intercostals. The internal intercostal muscles pull the ribs down and together pushing air out, and the external muscles have the opposite effect as they pull the ribs upwards. These can contribute as much as 15% of maximal airflow. When we are sedentary for long periods of time, the intercostal muscles need to do very little, so they become untrained, and even start to feel quite rigid.

Muscles in the front of the neck

The third and final group of primary muscles involved in breathing are the smallest and weakest of the three groups. They are located in the neck, and are known collectively as 'accessory muscles of the neck'. They act by lifting the first and second ribs, and can often be seen clearly as sinewy wires going down the side of the neck in people when they are struggling to breathe.

At maximal effort, the accessory muscles would only contribute up to 5% of the maximal airflow (see Figure 1.6). Healthy people usually recruit them only at times of real need, such as during high intensity activity. Oddly, this contrasts with the vast majority of the COPD patients I meet. It is common for these people to rely very heavily, sometimes almost entirely, on these small weak muscles for inhalation. Relying upon these small, insignificant muscles groups to drive respiration is a sign of breathing dysfunction and it is also very tiring. Not only do they fatigue very quickly, but they also tend to use up significant amounts of energy with very little effect on breathing efficiency.

The oxygen demand of breathing

The inefficient breathing patterns that COPD patients demonstrate mean that they can often be using between 50% and 70% of their energy expenditure just to drive respiration. This phenomenon may explain why some COPD patients become excessively thin, because their bodies are using up much of their energy intake simply to fuel their inefficient breathing. In comparison, a healthy person will use a negligible amount of energy to breathe, relying on the natural elasticity of the lungs and an open chest to provide the flow of air in and out of the lungs.

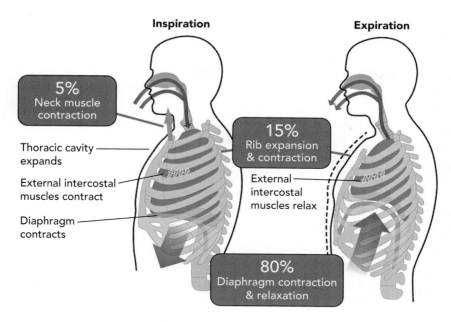

Inspiration

5%
Neck muscle
contraction

Thoracic cavity
expands

External intercostal
muscles contract

Diaphragm
contracts

15%
Rib expansion
& contraction

80%
Diaphragm contraction
& relaxation

Expiration

External
intercostal
muscles relax

Figure 1.6 *Approximate percentage contribution of the main muscle groups of respiration*

I have purposely simplified the number and extent of muscles involved in normal respiration to help you identify the way in which you breathe currently, and how you might be able to change this. There are a number of additional muscle groups that can influence inhalation and exhalation, especially during physical activity. You will not need to know these muscle groups and what they do to make use of this book, but if you want to read further into this, they are listed in Table 1.1.

Table 1.1: *Other muscles that have a part to play in respiration*

Inhalation	Exhalation
Latissimus dorsi (arms elevated)	Latissimus dorsi
Serratus anterior (arms elevated)	Abdominal muscles
Upper trapezius	Quadratus lumborum
Serratus posterior superior	Serratus posterior inferior
Sternocleidomastoid	

The most recent research done into the actions of the muscular system shows that the muscles do not work alone to provide the tension to move the skeleton and the body. There is another tissue that is understood to have profound effects on the postural positioning of the body in the static positions we adopt whilst at work or at rest. These tissues are known collectively as 'fascia'. Fascia is essentially connective tissue that helps to support and define the structure of muscles and organs, rather in the same way that the segments of an orange have distinct divisions. The fascia is thought to help take the strain of the muscles when they are overworked consistently over a long period of time. Fascia used to be called sinew. These structures are exceedingly strong and not only attach muscles to bone but can develop under the strains of gravity, caused in the main, by habitually poor posture. They tend to strengthen and tighten when we are inactive and when muscles are being continually overworked. This overuse is thought to cause the fascia to effectively become tight, leathery and dehydrated. The change in the structure of the fascia throughout the body, along with the muscular stiffness and joint rigidity that accompanies it, is thought to limit the natural flow of lymphatic fluids around the body, further increasing the incidence of discomfort or pain.

The control of breathing

Normally, breathing is automatic and subconscious for us all. The body does this by way of the autonomic nervous system. Our autonomic nervous system controls the rate and depth of our breathing, just as it controls other essential bodily functions like heart rate, blood flow, the endocrine system (hormonal), the transit of food through the digestive system, urination and sexual function. Autonomic control enables us to maintain a correct balance in the body from relaxed sleep, right the way through to the most vigorous forms of exercise.

The one time we will definitely have had to think about our breathing is when we have done an active sport or vigorous physical activity. Who remembers the burning-throat sensation of doing a school cross-country or another endurance-based sport that pushed us close to our physical limits? Others will think about the way in which they control their breathing when swimming, sequencing the breath with a stroke to prevent them sucking in water. The more musically minded may have played a wind instrument or sung, where breathing control was essential and required training and practice. Other than in these situations, very few of us continue to challenge our lungs mechanically over our extended lifetime.

In western societies, our modern way of living is becoming more and more sedentary. It is little surprise that most people who develop COPD only really become aware that they have a problem when they can't do simple daily tasks – tasks that have taken years or even decades to become an issue.

The rate and depth of our breathing are driven in the main by our body's balancing our blood pH, ensuring the correct levels of acid (oxygen) and alkali (carbon dioxide) are maintained. The lungs themselves have the ability to dilate the larger airways and this action of the smooth muscles around the airways is completely under autonomic nervous system control. The smooth muscles in the lung airways also have pressure receptors in them, and these can feed back directly to the brain informing us how pressurised our lungs are.

Fortunately, we are able to override the rate and depth of breathing by conscious effort, and this book will aim to show you how you can control your breathing in a variety of ways to engage your brain before you ask your body to do anything physically challenging.

Chapter 2

When breathing goes wrong

> ◊ **Shallow tidal breathing**
> ◊ **Conventional advice on breathing techniques**
> ◊ **Breathing problems – overbreathing**
> ◊ **Chest infections**
> ◊ **Other health problems – co-morbidities**

There are vast and varied ranges of factors that can set off an exacerbation of breathlessness. They can be almost instantaneous, or they can build up over time to create a considerable chronic breathing problem. These causal factors can be divided into three main groups – emotional, environmental and lifestyle-related, as summarised in Table 2.1.

Table 2.1: *Common contributing factors or triggers of breathlessness*

Emotional	Environmental	Lifestyle
Stress at home	Heat/humidity	Poor posture
Workload	Airborne pollutants	Poor exercise technique
Anxiety	Altitude	Sedentary lifestyle
Fear	Smoking	Poor health
Frustration	External air pressure	Poor diet

Each patient who presents at my clinic has their own story to tell about how their health has taken a turn for the worse. I try to look back at the sequence of events that may have contributed to their breathlessness as I find it can help them to understand that they are not always in a futile situation, but that they might be able to address some of the issues that have led them to breathe so poorly.

A typical, common example is when a patient has been forced to be inactive for a week or two. This might be due to a medical problem, such as illness or an accident, or it might be the length of time it has taken to recover from an operation unrelated to their lungs. This period of relative inactivity places minimal demand on major muscle groups, and they can soon become deconditioned. (I like to share an old adage to demonstrate this point: 'Seven days without exercise makes one weak.') The patient is usually totally oblivious to this deconditioning process and only becomes aware of the problem when they stand up and try to do something more active. At this point the new, limited breathing pattern the body has adopted can't cope.

Shallow tidal breathing

During normal quiet breathing the body's oxygen needs are limited in the main to powering the heart, brain, respiratory muscles and other vital organs. In healthy lungs, this quiet breathing would lead to approximately 500 ml of air moving in and out of the respiratory passages. Whilst 500 ml sounds like quite a lot, only about 300 ml of this air actually reaches the alveoli; the rest remains in the airways of the nose, pharynx, larynx, trachea, bronchi, and higher levels of the bronchioles. In contrast, COPD patients often take very shallow, rapid breaths that take in much less air with each breath. To compensate for this restricted intake of air, the body automatically responds by speeding up the breathing rate. You may recognise the feeling of panting and wheezing as the air is sucked into a very tight chest. It feels like the airways are being scrunched up, and in fact that is exactly what is happening.

A COPD patient who is breathing poorly can be taking in as little as 300 ml every time they pant. As with the healthy lung, the first 200 ml remains in the upper airways. This means that the COPD patient maybe functioning on as little as 100 ml of air in the alveoli, considerably less than the body would need for any form of physical activity. Often the amount of oxygen on supply is only enough for the basic body functions, like breathing, digestion and the heart muscle pumping. Regularly, I meet a patient who is taking in so little air from panting, that they can hardly focus their mind on what I am talking to them about.

When the quantity of air reaching the lungs is so scarce, and with such short periods of time in the lungs, there is little chance for adequate oxygenation of the bloodstream. Blood chemoreceptors react to these lower levels of oxygen by telling the brain to further increase the rate of breathing. This feedback loop can soon become extremely stressful. Not only can it lead to a feeling of discomfort, anxiety and fear, but if it happens suddenly or intensely it can cause extreme panic.

Panic breathing

Worse is still to come. When you panic, your body then fights ever more desperately to inhale. The desperate inhalation becomes very taxing and, over time, the patient develops a chronic, active inhalation technique, something that is not only wasteful of energy but also utterly exhausting and stressful. This is sometimes described as 'over-breathing syndrome' or 'hyperventilation syndrome'.

Conventional advice on breathing techniques

When I was taught about breathing, every physiology book I read explained the process of breathing through a healthy lung, within a healthy normal body. Inhalation was always explained as an active process, with the dome of the diaphragm contracting, drawing down into the space between the lungs and the abdominal area, and sucking the air into the body. Exhalation was always explained as a passive process, with the diaphragm relaxing and the lungs returning to their original size under their own elasticity. It has always been assumed that this is the same process for everybody, but I have found that at the ends of the fitness spectrum, where the body has adapted to particular physical demands, the normal process may differ slightly.

I believe that, like most things to do with physical capacity, there is no one-size-fits-all approach, and we need to personalise the programme as much as possible to help each individual. In my work with COPD patients I have found that the vast majority of these patients have one or more habitual issue that prevents the 'traditionally accepted' normal breathing pattern from taking place effectively. I have even found focusing on inhalation/inspiration causes some COPD patients to over-breathe, especially when they have been so used to sucking air in actively.

When I coach people, I have an aversion to anything that makes a patient feel under pressure, stressed or anxious, so I find focusing on active inhalation at all costs counter-productive. From working with patients, I quickly observed that they could inhale more passively given the right cues. I then had to develop a simple explanation that could prove my point. This is a key element of the Brice Method and will be explored at length throughout this book.

Probably the most widely used active inhalation technique, that is currently taught, is that of 'abdominal breathing' (see Figure 2.1). This is also known as 'diaphragmatic breathing', and is designed to help patients focus on drawing air in to the lungs by pushing the tummy forwards, allowing the diaphragm and lungs to drop into the space vacated by the moving gut in the abdominal cavity. I used to use this technique extensively for people with asthma and people who were overweight, but very quickly found that COPD patients often struggled to get the air in because of factors that other groups of people did not have to overcome.

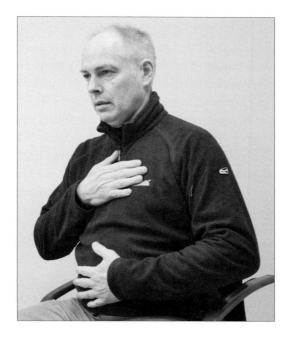

Figure 2.1 *Abdominal breathing technique*

Abdominal breathing training is the traditional teaching method used for COPD sufferers. You will find this on most websites and in most books, focusing on using the forward movement of the abdominal mass to assist the diaphragm to actively suck air into the lungs.

I started to try and find an alternative method of breathing training, one that would not make my patients feel uncomfortable, or appear so stressed. I soon realised that it was less important to help the patients strengthen and activate their diaphragms than it was to help give them more space in their lungs so that the diaphragm could work efficiently. Working concertedly with numerous patients, I found that they did not need to focus on active IN-halation, but to work more on active EX-halation. My patients immediately started to show that by controlling their exhalation, they were calmer, their breathing rate was slower, and they were breathing more deeply. The benefits of active exhalation will be an important theme throughout this book.

Breathing problems

Most, but not all, people with COPD have been smokers at some time in their lives. This fact remains, even though it is not productive to focus on it, as it cannot be undone. I do, however, believe that most smokers adopt a different breathing pattern from the rest of us. You just need to watch a smoker take a drag on a cigarette to see this could be the case. In my experience, almost all smokers appear to have trained themselves to use the sinew-like muscles of the neck to draw in the cigarette smoke. I believe that this sucking pattern of breathing soon becomes habitual. If you find that you tend to predominantly use your neck muscles when you breathe, this might be one of the factors that contributed to you adopting this modified breathing pattern in the first place. You can unlearn this 'sucking in hard' habit, and this will be covered in the exercises later.

Over-breathing

As a COPD sufferer, it is likely that you will recognise how easy it is to find yourself over-breathing at the slightest degree of exertion. Over-breathing is sometimes called hyperventilation, and it is not exclusively the result of physical activity. There are a number of psychological issues that can bring on hyperventilation, most of which originate around the feelings of fear, frustration or embarrassment. Over-breathing, can also be caused by physiological 'red flags', such as low levels of blood carbon dioxide. The concept that low levels of carbon dioxide can increase the rate and depth of breathing may sound a little strange at first, primarily because we might think that it is low levels of oxygen that might be the main driver of breathing rate and depth. Rather than look into this now, I have included a section on hyperventilation syndrome in Chapter 10 (page 130).

Over-breathing during physical activity

To help patients understand how they might be causing themselves to over-breathe when they first start exercising, I use a very basic description of how the lungs react to having high, or low, pressures inside them.

The lungs have stretch receptors in the smooth muscle of the bronchi and bronchioles (look back to Figure 1.3), which help gauge how empty or full the lungs are. For simplicity's sake, I tell patients that their lungs send warning signals if they inflate to within 15% of their normal maximum level, and similarly warn if they deflate to within 15% of their normal minimum level. Thus, if you breathe in too deeply, the lungs will react by actively contracting to force air out quickly and forcibly. If we assume a healthy lung has 100% capacity, there is a range of 70% capacity remaining once you take the 15% warning zone at each end of the spectrum (30% in total), so a single, over-deep breath has plenty of space to work within and it unlikely to cause too much air to be expelled from the lung too quickly (see Figure 2.2).

If a COPD patient has 30% damage to their lungs (shown grey in Figure 2.2), this means they only have 40% capacity that they can comfortably breathe before the lungs send warning signals to increase breathing rate and depth.

I teach my patients not to breathe in or out too deeply, keeping them out of their stress zones.

Chest infections

The lungs are a warm, moist environment, and are a perfect breeding ground for bacteria and infections. When a bug gets into a healthy set of lungs, the lining of the lung cell walls produces mucus to help catch and collect the bug so that it can be forced out under the pressure and flow of normal exhalation. This is assisted by tiny hair-like structures called cilia that are found in the larger airways, that act to waft the bug up and out of the lung to be coughed up. This warm, wet mucus is pretty much

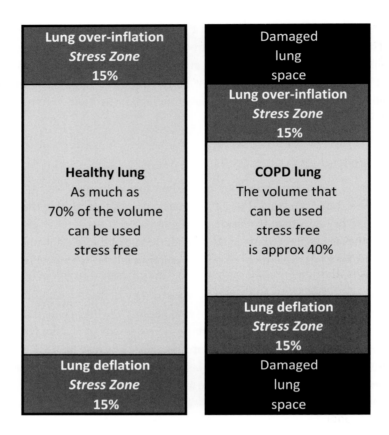

Figure 2.2: *Depth of inhalation and exhalation in healthy versus COPD lungs*

the exact same environment a biochemist would replicate if they wanted to breed their own bacteria in the lab. They use a gel with a bug in a petri dish, keep it warm and, as this will speed up the bug's metabolism, it grows at an accelerated rate.

The human body is designed to clear out bugs from the lungs, as well as mucus, by allowing air to move deeply in and out of the lungs. Nowadays, one of the main problems appears to be that the human body was not designed to be so inactive. For millions of years the structure and function of the human body have evolved as a result of constant, varied physical activity. Today's relatively inactive lifestyle means our bodies are quickly becoming accustomed to our lungs having very little to do. Is it any wonder such a neglect is having a negative impact on our lives, especially as we are now generally living longer than we used to?

Armed with this knowledge, I challenge my patients to choose between either doing nothing physically and relying upon medication to prevent the symptoms of breathlessness occurring, or being more active and helping their body deal with the cause. It may sound harsh, but it is true.

Other health problems – co-morbidities

More often than not, patients will present to me with one or more co-morbidities. Co-morbidities are other health conditions that a patient will have when they present at clinic. I will discuss these other health issues right at the start of their first consultation, as the answers give me an insight into what may have contributed to their becoming so breathless, as is illustrated by Margaret's case (see box).

***

Case study – Margaret

Margaret had COPD and very painful knees, with limited range of motion, so it was difficult for her to stand up. She had to wait a year to have replacement knee surgery and she admitted that she had been less active than usual prior to the surgery due to the pain. Margaret's recovery from the knee surgery was slow, and her family helped her out, so she found she was just as inactive for the two years following the surgery. Being sedentary for a prolonged period of time, Margaret put on weight and ended up slumped on the sofa, or slumped in bed. By being less active, Margaret's body had learned to cope with the lessened demand for oxygen, and her breathing pattern altered by becoming shallower and more rapid. Once Margaret tried to exercise, the newly formed breathing pattern could not cope with the increased oxygen demand of walking to the loo.

Margaret's breathlessness meant she was referred to me for exercise.

***

Whilst patients may be referred to me specifically to treat their COPD, a significant number of them will have co-morbidities that are potentially more limiting than their impaired breathing. It is very common to have problems associated with musculo-skeletal disease, injuries that are the result of accidents, or hereditary complaints that prevent a person from doing certain movements. In these situations, the type of pain that they feel may be extremely debilitating. For these patients, I have to ensure that before they start to exercise, they understand what feelings of discomfort or pain are realistic for them to have to put up with as they start and eventually progress through their programme of exercises. The way in which people identify and describe pain is key to helping them understand the difference between, say, discomfort, good pain and bad pain. Pain tolerance is a very personal thing, and whilst some people will have low threshold for pain naturally, others will carry on oblivious to any feeling whatsoever. Low pain threshold can be due to a patient simply being hypersensitive to pain, or it can even be that they are anticipating that something will be as painful as it has been previously, and it becomes a self-fulfilling prophecy.

Regaining joint movement

Rather like the hinges on an unused car door, an inactive human joint can become 'rusty'. The amazing thing about the human body is that, unlike a car door, human joints are self-lubricating, and can, with time, regain much of their mobility. I have seen numerous octogenarians regain 20 years' worth of exercise capacity, with small numbers of repetitions of extremely simple and gentle movements.

It is possible for a patient to report unexpectedly high levels of pain for a gentle activity simply because it is a sensation that they have never experienced before. This pain may be related to their lung condition, or it may be linked to one or more other co-morbidities. Those people who have experienced pain in the past will often anticipate its onset and their bodies learn to over-compensate by flinching, or recruiting other muscle groups as an automatic reflex to try and stop the pain from being repeated. Low back pain is a common example of a situation where pain that is not linked to the lungs can limit a patient's ability to exercise and adversely affect their breathing. For some patients, even the slightest sign of pain in the low back will cause a reflex spasm of supporting muscles, further reducing the ability of the body to move freely, and potentially increasing the level of pain with continued movement. Unfortunately, muscle spasms such as these can cause people to react by holding their breath. This breath hold is a particularly common outcome when the pain is relatively severe. I have included a guide to how you can differentiate between good pain and bad pain in the Introduction (page 8).

The shape, movement and location of the rib cage all play a pivotal part in the proper functioning of the lungs. This is why the first exercises I give people are ones that help them to be aware of and improve their posture, and these are the subject of Chapter 3.

Chapter 3

Postural self-awareness

◊   Kyphosis – How slumping adversely affects breathing

1.   Your head acts like a yoke around your neck

2.   Slumping causes your shoulders to hang forwards

3.   Slumping concertinas your ribs together

4.   Slumping pushes your diaphragm onto your belly

◊ Posture really matters

As a trained exercise physiologist, I always return to my grounding that the most profound and constant limiting factor for human performance is gravity. Whilst it may not be obvious why gravity might have a key role in the way in which we breathe, it is the one force that is always present whatever we are doing and wherever we are, and the way our bodies react against gravity gives us our own very personal posture.

I would estimate that more than 95% of the people I meet in my clinic present with poor breathing patterns that can be directly linked to poor posture. Most of the time they have their head held in a forward position. This body position is known as 'kyphosis' (see Figure 3.1).

Kyphosis can be the result of one of many lifestyle issues. Lots of older patients I work with have had plenty of time to accumulate other health conditions that can have

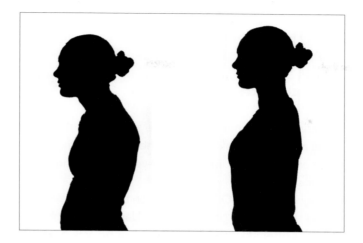

Figure 3.1: *Kyphosis and erect posture – side view*

contributed to them adopting a slumped position. Some have spent so much of their retired life inactive, either slumped on a sofa or lying in bed, that they find they get stuck in that slumped rut. In western society we are becoming more and more sedentary in our work; our recreational activities are also less active than they used to be, and these are important factors that contribute to a hunched body position. Poor posture can also be an inherited trait. Have you ever noticed how families will often walk with the children showing similar movement patterns to one of their parents? Some of this may be down to nature, but some will be down to nurture, as children tend to learn by copying their parents' movement patterns from an early age.

I have coached lots of sports people, and the ones who slouch the most are the young rowers. Long levers help in rowing, so many of them are extremely tall. Being considerably taller than their peers, they may feel they have to stoop to fit in with their friends at school; some even have stoop to physically fit under a normal doorway without banging their heads. There are also skeletal conditions such as ankylosing spondilitis, scoliosis or osteoporosis, that can affect a person's postural structure. Or it could be due to a trauma, such as a road traffic accident, that has weakened the neck. Everyone has his or her own background story that needs to be borne in mind.

I myself am not immune to the head-forwards posture, and recognise that I tend to slump when I use my laptop, tablet or mobile phone for any length of time.

Case study – watchmaker

I remember a career watchmaker in his late seventies, who had spent nearly 50 years bent over, looking at watches for more than 10 hours a day. When he came in he would have his eyes on my shoes, whether he was standing or sitting.

He was diagnosed with COPD at Level 4 on the MRC scale (see page 3), and he was also taking eight paracetamol a day for his kyphotic back pain. Three weeks after starting the programme he was down to three paracetamol a week and finding breathing much less problematic.

He put this down to the fact that he did daily exercises that forced him to be aware of his posture, and even though he was extraordinarily slumped, he got a relatively quick reduction in pain.

A month later he was totally off the painkillers and could look me in the eye. When I pointed it out to him that he could see me above my waist, he laughed and told me I wasn't as good looking as my female colleague! That is gratitude for you.

How slumping adversely affects breathing

I have found that to help persuade my patients not to sit or stand with their heads leaning forward I need to explain how this body position can prevent them from breathing properly. Whilst not everyone sits forwards noticeably, probably 95% of my patients slump to some degree or another.

Your head acts like a yoke round your neck

Being in kyphosis, the body has to work actively against gravity to stop the head from lolling forwards, and as a result the muscles that hold the head upright in the back of the neck have to work extra hard (see Figure 3.2). Holistic practitioners, body workers and manual therapists of all kinds look for a degree of balance and harmony in the body. When you see a person with an upright posture (see the left-hand image on the sequence in Figure 3.2), the head looks like it is balanced on top of the spine. The muscles in the neck are under approximately 5 kg of pressure, so there is little tension to make the individual feel tight or stressed. This person looks at ease.

This is in stark contrast to the slumped individual shown on the far right of Figure 3.2, where the neck and upper back muscles have to work extremely hard to prevent the head from lolling forwards.

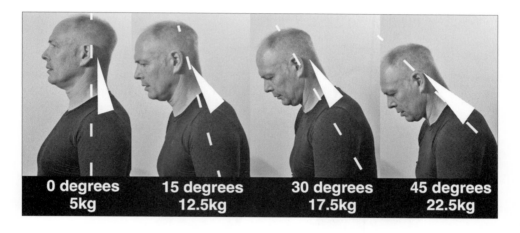

Figure 3.2: *Relative strain on neck muscles, with head forward position*

I usually explain this mechanism by taking a side-on picture of my patients and comparing it to Figure 3.2. I explain how each position is like having a heavy yoke hanging round your neck, all day, every day! As the head slumps further forward the force the neck muscles have to exert increases considerably. I am quite strong, but lifting a 22.5 kg dumbbell on to the desk, and thudding it down, is very sobering. Showing patients how much strain their neck is under if they hold their head at 45 degrees from the shoulder, they tend to listen more intently to what I have to tell them next.

Additionally, if a patient adopts this body position for any length of time, it can lead to a relative shortening of the muscles at the rear of the neck as they take the strain of the weight of the head. At its most overused and extreme form, it is thought that this shortening of the neck muscles can even pinch the phrenic nerves, as they originate

41

from between the 2nd to 6th cervical vertebrae of the spine. The phrenic nerves drive the muscular action of the diaphragm, and there is the possibility that the forward head position may inhibit the normal control of the diaphragm.

Slumping causes your shoulders to hang forwards

The head-forwards position usually results in the shoulder blades being lifted and drawn forwards around the upper ribs, hanging forward and downwards in relation to the ribcage (see Figure 3.3). This causes further loading on the postural muscles of the neck. This relentless loading compresses downwards on the rib cage, rather like the weight of the world being on your shoulders.

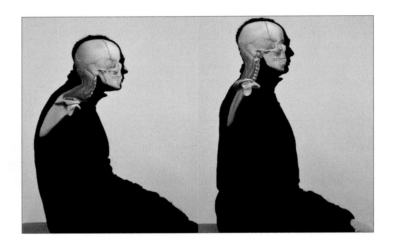

Figure 3.3 *Slumped shoulder blades versus upright shoulder carriage*

While the shoulders are hanging forwards, the small muscle groups at the front of the neck are usually simultaneously tightened and shortened. This can be to the point where the vocal chords are affected by the resulting tension in the throat and upper chest. The breath that accompanies this kyphotic body positioning is usually shallow and rapid and, with even the slightest physical demand, the limited air flow leads to an even more rapid and shorter breath.

Demonstrating the effect of shoulders hanging forwards

If you do not think that you are affected by this problem, or you have a family member who does not understand how it feels to not breathe very well, you might like to know of an exercise I teach other medics. I do this to get across the importance of posture on breathing. This is described in Figure 3.4 below.

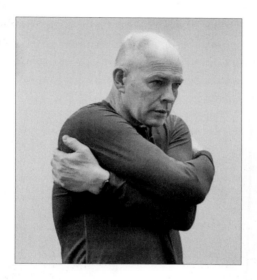

Figure 3.4: *Straitjacket demonstration*
1. *Imagine you are in a straitjacket, and you have people pulling your arms across your body so that your elbows cross in front of you.*
2. *Reach your hands as far round your back as possible, holding your shoulder blades with your fingers.*
3. *Breathe out as deeply as you can, readjusting your hands so that you can tightly grip your shoulder blades.*
4. *Maintain your hands in this position.*
5. *Now try and breathe in deeply!*

Inevitably, when you assume this 'straitjacket' posture, a deep and satisfying inhalation is nigh on impossible, as the lungs have nowhere to expand into.

Slumping concertinas your ribs together

The loading of the head and shoulders pushes down on the rib cage, causing the intercostal muscles between the ribs to shorten (see Figure 3.5), and over time they can lose much of their natural elasticity. Eventually, under continued loading, they learn to play no part in normal respiration. In extreme cases, a patient's chest will appear to be concave, with the sternum (the cartilage that runs down the front of the rib cage) drawn back towards the spine and downward towards the pelvis. It is little wonder that this person cannot get a satisfying inhalation.

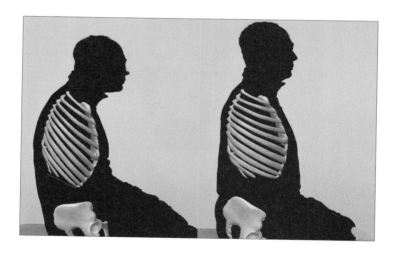

Figure 3.5: *Slumped and concertina-ed ribs versus upright, open rib cage*

Even if you are very strong, and gravity is not the force that causes you to slump, there are other potential reasons why you might adopt this posture when you have COPD. Rather like a hedgehog, we humans have a natural reaction to curl up when we feel desperately endangered. Not being able to breathe is one of the most stressful things that we can endure. The feeling of suffocation you get when you have a COPD exacerbation is so great, is it little wonder that the resulting uncontrollable panic makes sufferers want to curl up in the foetal position to get some relief? Again, over time this can become an automatic reaction to the stress of breathlessness that immediately leads to the intercostal muscles contracting.

I want my patients to become aware that they are not moving their chest, and how if we can coax these muscles back into action, they can regain mobility, and once more play an active part in respiration.

Slumping pushes your diaphragm onto your belly

As the diaphragm acts like a muscular skirt across the bottom of the rib cage, the slumped upper body pushes down, fixing the diaphragm in place on top of the intestinal mass (see Figure 3.6). In some patients (especially those who have been on multiple steroid treatments) the intestinal mass has become quite bloated, making this situation even worse.

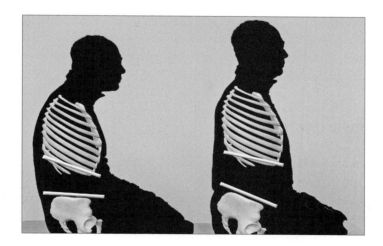

Figure 3.6: *Slumped belly versus supportive and toned abdominals*

With the ribcage depressed so that the whole weight of the upper body is pushing down onto the abdomen, the diaphragm is unable to work as it is designed to. Normally, in a balanced body, the diaphragm should be lifted off the intestines and tensioned by the open rib cage; this leaves a pressure gradient between the upper body and the lower body for the diaphragm to draw downwards with little resistance on inhalation. If you remember, a healthy individual gets approximately 75% of their resting tidal volume from the action of the diaphragm. Slumping forwards and preventing the diaphragm contracting is possibly the most profound effect of the kyphotic posture.

It is interesting to note that a good percentage of my COPD patients get acid reflux or have a diagnosis of hiatus hernia. To me it is little surprise that they get this reflux of stomach contents travelling up the oesophagus, as downward pressure on the stomach from a compressed diaphragm could potentially cause this to happen. Most of my patients have said that their symptoms of reflux have either reduced or disappeared after following the Brice Method. This is not something I can claim responsibility for, but it would be interesting to do some further research on this effect.

A further issue that can be linked to the diaphragm being pushed down onto the belly is an impaired lymphatic flow. The lymphatic system is rather like the body's sewage system, and it is very reliant upon the action of the diaphragm to allow the system to work effectively. With the diaphragm caught between the overly pressurised lungs and heavily pressurised gut, it may contribute to the pooling of waste products around the body and the sluggishness of lymphatic flow. This can lead to a patient experiencing fatigue, malaise and even pain.

Posture really matters

I hope you have taken the time to understand this chapter about the benefits of healthy posture.

I try to give as persuasive an argument to my patients as I can to convince them that they *must* try to adopt an open chest posture because otherwise they will always struggle to reach their full breathing potential.

I strongly believe that you must first address postural issues *before* you try to improve your breathing technique and before you start the Brice Method exercise programme.

Chapter 4

Learning to de-slump yourself

Now that you have read about the potential pitfalls of slumping and how it might be one of the crucial factors that limits your breathing, I will share with you the first and possibly the most vital exercise that you will do within the Brice Method. Please don't be tempted to skip mastering this, thinking it is too basic to pay any real attention to. It is simple but can have profound benefits if you pay full attention to the details included. That, along with practice, may be one of the most important skills you can learn from this book.

Being aware of your body and actively de-slumping is a key skill that you will be asked to repeat before you undertake any activity, even going to the toilet!

De-slumping exercise

Preparation

For this exercise, you will need a high-backed chair that is firm and supportive. You will find a sofa or lounge chair will be far too soft to provide any meaningful support to your spine. A dining table chair with arms or a relatively firm office chair is what you will need. If the chair has arms, it may assist you, but if your chair has no arms you can still do the exercise.

You will also need a rolled-up towel or a back support of some sort draped over the top of the backrest (see Figure 4.1). A description of the different types of back support you can use is detailed in Addendum 2 (page 141), but to start, a rolled-up towel should suffice.

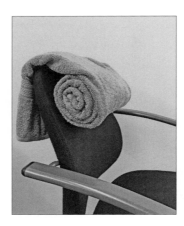

Figure 4.1: *Rolled-up towel back support*

Self-awareness preparation

Sit on a chair as you normally would. Position a rolled-up towel or back support as shown on the right-hand side of Figure 4.2 (supported posture) and listen again to your breathing as you did before in the Landmark 1 Self-test earlier in the book (page 13).

Ask yourself the following questions and be more aware of what you are actually doing when you inhale and exhale:

- notice where your head is in relation to your body

48

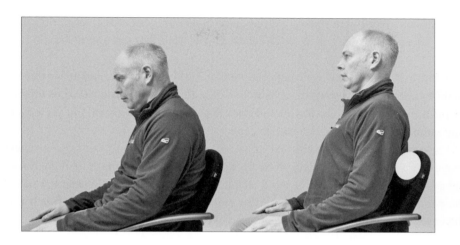

Figure 4.2: *Unsupported versus supported posture*

- notice how you are holding your shoulders
- think about the pace and speed of your breathing
- recognise how deep your breath is going into your lungs
- think about how satisfying each breath is.

How to do the exercise

- Sit down on the firm high-backed chair, with your bottom pushed right back into the seat.
- Ensure that the rolled-up towel or back support pad is positioned below and between your shoulder blades (refer back to Figure 4.2). The rolled-up towel or pad should be big enough for you to feel it push against your ribs, but not so big that you are being toppled forwards.
- Now try to draw your shoulder blades backwards and downwards, whilst drawing the nape of your neck backwards. The towel or back support will act as a pivot point, allowing your ribs to open up like a fan, and artificially supporting and expanding your chest in the process.
- When you draw your shoulders backwards and downwards, you may find that your hands will need to fall by your hips or slide back on the arms of your

49

chair. Work with this by putting your hands on your hips if your chair has no arms, or drawing your elbows back if your chair has got arm rests.

Some lucky individuals (a rough estimate of 35%) will get immediate improvement in their breathlessness from this position. While the head lifts and balances on the top of the spine, the shoulder blades fall back into a relaxed position and the ribs flare open; the lungs expand inside the rib cage.

For most, this position will feel quite odd at first as you are asking your chest to move in a way it may not have done for some considerable time. The body does not always like change, especially rapid change, so please take a little time to relax into the position gradually. A few may even feel the position is rather painful. If this is the case for you, don't force things too quickly, but please persevere; many a patient who would have given up after feeling a little odd at this stage has gone on to surprise me with the considerable improvements they have made in their breathing over the programme.

At first this new body alignment is challenging the posture that you may have developed over months, years or possibly even decades, so it won't be corrected overnight. In reality, most patients take a little time to let the body settle down and recognise that this new posture is not wrong for them. It is just different. When your body has got used to being held in one position for a long time, it is essentially 'stuck in a rut', and getting out of that rut needs some determined and repeated effort.

As your back continues to press against the towel, or pad, below and between your shoulder blades, it will directly push against your ribs. As your ribs are directly attached to your spine, you may notice that as your body relaxes that your head lifts and you feel as if you have become taller. This elongation of the body may mean that you start to feel the muscles around your waist work a little harder. (Engaging the muscles of your waist is part of the body's natural balancing mechanism, and later on in the book you will discover how it aids natural breathing – see page 84.)

Moving yourself into a more erect position can feel a little unnatural at first; you may even find that your body will tell you it does not like it. Most of my patients have been so slumped for so long that their body has got used to being in a poor posture. If you do feel uncomfortable in this new position, rest assured that this should only be temporary, and your discomfort should ease away relatively quickly. (Refer back to the monitoring any pain section in the Introduction.) Holding this upright position for a few minutes can help take some of the strain off the muscles that are normally holding you slumped forwards. Again, you may feel some neck discomfort, but if you can try to relax and persevere, you are likely to find some relief as the body moulds to its more erect stance. I joke with my patients to help them realise that having a little discomfort is natural. I tell them that their rib cage is used to being as flexible as a breezeblock, and will take a little while to recognise that it can move again. Whilst it is a lame joke, a smile can often help reduce tension. So, the advice here is, don't try to push it or force it; let it happen naturally. There is a song title there methinks!

If you are one of the lucky ones, who immediately find their body falling onto a position of ease, with their head feeling balanced on top of their neck, the muscles of their neck and upper shoulders feeling slack and relaxed, and their chest falling open, you will begin to realise that your breathing is no longer driven by your neck muscles. You may even find that you do not need to suck air in as much.

Advice if you have back problems
If you have a severe back problem that means you cannot use a direct support against your ribs, you can alternatively try to perch on the front of a chair keeping your spine as upright as possible, with your shoulders drawn back and your head retracted over your body. This is very similar to the position you would otherwise adopt in the Brice Method.

The standing alternative

There is an alternative approach if you do not have a suitable chair, or if you get severe pain in the back from doing the de-slumping exercise sitting down.

You can do this exercise standing up against a wall if you prefer. To do this you will need to stand with your back to the wall, with your feet about 10 inches (25 cm) away from the wall and with your knees very slightly bent. This bend in the knees helps to stop the pelvis from rocking forwards and engages the tummy muscles slightly. The towel or support pad needs to be between you and the wall in exactly the same place as shown in Figure 4.2, and you will need to follow the instructions as if you were seated, keeping your knees slightly bent and your hips not tilted forwards. Leaning back against the support towards the wall will open up your rib cage in the same way it did in the seated position.

Having the support of the pad behind your back has the effect of pushing your rib cage forwards, upwards and flaring it outwards. Your spine simultaneously regains a more erect position, causing your head to draw up and back over your body and taking some of the strain off your neck.

The amount of improvement to your posture will depend upon the degree of immobility that you have had, the length of time you have been slumped, plus any other conditions that contribute to your discomfort. Do, however, try to persevere with this exercise; it will play a pivotal part in your progression, and failure to improve this will greatly limit your progress through the remainder of this book.

What to do if you are feeling light-headed and woozy
Every so often, I get patients who feel slightly woozy or light-headed just from adopting this erect body position. If you do get this problem, it is likely that, over time, you have developed such a forced inhalation technique from breathing that you will habitually try to suck maximum amounts of air into your chest, even when your body does not need it. As this new body position opens up your chest, negating the need to actively suck the air in hard, the chest is pretty much full, and you will feel like you are over-breathing. Over-breathing in this situation can be rather distressing, but do not worry overly about this; you will learn later in the book some techniques to overcome this issue.

Fine-tuning the position of the back support

The positioning of the back support between you and the chair or wall will ultimately depend upon personal preference. I recommend that you start with the gentler option of the towel or spongy roll, as these provide you with enough support to relax your body and breathe deeply with less direct pressure than the other options that I will detail later. The towel and the pad tend to give a generalised effect, working over a number of ribs.

The best location for the towel or lumber roll is just below the lower point of your shoulder blades, closest to your spine. This will give support and provide a pivot in the middle of your back as the forward pressure is placed between four and six ribs at a time. This is shown as position C in Figure 4.3. As the supports are quite large and will not fit between the shoulder blades easily, many of my patients find that they progress on to spikey peanuts or tennis balls placed in a sock. These supports are smaller and firmer, and push against the rib cage to open one to three ribs at a time. As such, they are ideal to open up specific areas of the chest. (See Addendum 2, page 142, for more details on these types of equipment.)

In Figure 4.3, you can see the vertical placement of three smaller, more direct supports: A, B and C.

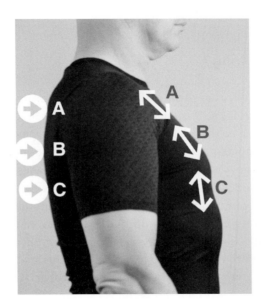

Figure 4.3 *Location of support*

A.   *If you place the support high between the shoulder blades you will find the top part of the rib cage will open up if you lean back against the support.*

B.   *Supporting mid-way down the rib cage, between the lowest corner of the shoulder blades, will open the mid region of the rib cage.*

C.   *Supports on the lower ribs, below the shoulder blades, will flare open the lowest part of the rib cage.*

In complete contrast to the general effects of the towel and the lumbar role, the tennis balls or spikey peanuts will need much more trial and error to best suit your body.

Using these tools not only helps you gain self-awareness, but as you try the ball in different places you will find that place where you get the most ease. The experience of being aware of your lungs and how you can improve your breathing by doing something as simple as this can be quite liberating.

As you practise the exercise above you will get more accustomed to using the back support. Over time your body may eventually change shape, and you may find that you need to alter the position of the support to get the most benefit.

How often, how long?

I recommend that you first try to sit in this position four or five times each day. The main reason for doing this so frequently, especially in the first few weeks, is so that you start to recognise how the relative positioning of your spine, head, shoulders and ribs plays such an important part in how you can breathe more naturally. Regular practice is the only way you will break old habits. Old habits tend to die hard, but regular, consistent effort almost always works for my patients.

You can adopt this position for as long as you feel comfortable. That might be for a minute before you have to stop, or you may be able to maintain the position for a maximum of about 10 minutes before it becomes uncomfortable. How long you keep the support in place is entirely up to you. Remember that if you do feel even a moderate amount of pain, you are unlikely to get the benefit of relaxed breathing you are aiming for. If you suffer from arthritis and get severe pain in the neck or shoulders when you do this exercise, either reposition yourself so you can lower the pain level, or leave the exercise a little while until you can try it again and remain relatively pain free. (Remember, you can always refer to the section on monitoring pain in the Introduction, page 8.)

As you practise the upright, de-slumped posture you will find that your lungs are opened up naturally. You will find that air is drawn into your lungs without the need to actively inhale. This may feel quite surprising, even quite unnerving at first. If you have spent the last few months or years trying to force air into a compressed lung by sucking, you will probably be amazed at how easy it is to inhale in this position. With practice, your body should be able to regulate the amount of air it takes in passively, only taking in the amount it needs to do a certain activity. This is precisely what the human body was designed to do! When you get used to sitting and standing like this you may find that slumping in your sofa, and leaning over counter tops become your lungs' worst enemies. Your upright pose should hopefully become your new 'position of ease'.

For most of my patients who are able to learn this erect breathing technique, there is not any real need to train muscles of inhalation. Inhalation training is the mainstay of most rehabilitation programmes; however, I feel that this technique becomes pretty much redundant. I would even go as far as to say that active inhalation training at the early stages of breathing training is counter-productive as it emphasises hard work, often recruiting the neck muscles when they are not needed, and most importantly overlooks the significance of having an open chest and lungs. I feel that inhalation training should only really be used for COPD patients once they are able to breathe in a relaxed fashion and are starting to get fit enough to extend themselves into what might be considered full fitness training.

Tracking your progress

Once you feel that you have managed to experience some benefit from Exercise 1, do the Landmark 2 Self-test which follows this chapter, and then move straight on to the following chapters, as executing the next few exercises is likely to help mobilise your upper body and facilitate your adopting a more upright posture.

Landmark 2

At this stage you should re-do the self-test that you did before you started reading Chapter 1 of this book.

Self-test 2

Take a deep breath, and think about where you can feel the air inside your body. Draw on the picture of the torso below where you feel the air going in your body.

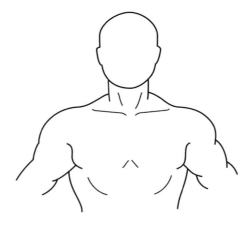

Once you have drawn the full extent of where you feel the air go into your chest, I would like you to note down how you would rate the quality of this breath on a scale of 1 to 10.

1	2	3	4	5	6	7	8	9	10
Poor				Average			Good		Fantastic

Check your scoring and compare this with Self-test 1 that you did at Landmark 1 (page 13). See if your score has improved.

Chapter 5

Relaxed breathing techniques

◊   Visualisation exercise – spongy lungs

◊   Exhalation – the driving force of breathing for the COPD lungs

◊   Pursed-lip breathing

◊   Pacing and timing

      Parachute counting

      Paced breathing

◊   Inhalation muscle training

◊   Pros and cons of nasal breathing

◊   Abdominal breathing

◊   Are you ready to progress?

On average I see more than 200 new patients a year, either walking in or being wheeled in, totally oblivious to the fact that they can have some control over the way that they breathe. The majority of these patients come into my clinic working desperately hard to suck in air against a compressed chest and lungs. Whilst I am quickly able to show them that posture has a big part to play in the amount and ease with which air can be inhaled, I find many have been taught techniques that are not always specifically designed for COPD patients.

When I started working with large numbers of COPD patients I suddenly realised that most of the breathing techniques they had been recommended differed very little from standard breathing techniques used for the general population with healthy lungs, or for asthma sufferers.

If you take time to look on the Internet, in COPD advice booklets, there are usually four breathing techniques that are recommended as a standard. They are:
1. pursed-lip breathing
2. inhalation muscle training
3. nasal breathing
4. abdominal breathing.

Of these four techniques, only one actually focuses on exhalation (pursed lip breathing); the other three highlight inhalation exercises.

From our de-slumping exercise, you should hopefully recognise that the lungs can be opened up pretty easily, and this is why I tend to shy away from the inhalation training techniques, especially at the start of the programme when I am trying to instil relaxed, quiet and comfortable breathing techniques. I find the inhalation training techniques tend to aggravate the situation, as the emphasis is on breathing in hard, and controlling breathing in a forceful way, all of which tend to make my patients more, not less, stressed!

To get this message across to my patients clearly, I use a simple visual exercise to show how the lungs work when you are breathing. The exercise usually sticks in the mind once you have seen it because it is so obvious. Whilst it could be seen as a vast over-simplification of the process of breathing, it is more pertinent to most patients with COPD than you would at first think.

Visualisation exercise – spongy lungs

I use a big sponge that is about the same size as my lungs – see Figure 5.1. When you breathe in, your shoulders are drawn back and down, which opens your rib cage and lifts it off your belly. Inside your chest your lungs are like sponges that are also open, with plenty of air in them. It takes relatively little effort to get the air in, as the spongy lung is expanded automatically.

Then I squeeze the sponge and breathe out slowly, showing them that the air should flow out easily and without too much effort. As I expand my chest and draw my

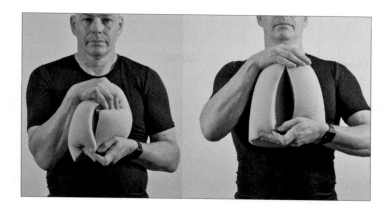

Figure 5.1: *Spongy lung demonstration*

shoulders back again, I release the sponge and it pings open, just like the lungs will do if the chest is kept open.

I ask patients to imagine they are breathing along with me as I repeat the exercise. I get them to think that they are breathing out slowly as I constrict the sponge, blowing through pursed lips to slow down and regulate the flow of air.

I repeat this a few times, asking patients to follow my lead and making sure they don't suck in too hard. If they do breathe as they habitually would and suck in lots of air, I warn them that they will almost certainly feel 'light headed', as the body is quickly over-oxygenated. As mentioned in previous chapters, the body wants the chemistry of the blood to be in balance: too much oxygen is just as bad as too little.

I explain how these deeper breaths are drawing air right into the air sacs, rather than simply flowing up and down the larger pipes of the lungs.

With practice, patients tell me they find this new breathing technique very relaxing. The lungs rebound open and the in-breath just seems to happen naturally. Because the rib cage is lifted off the abdominal mass, the diaphragm can work unhindered without having to try and force the belly out of the way as it descends. The intercostal muscles between the ribs are free to do their thing, lifting and separating if a deeper breath is needed. With time, the neck muscles no longer have to be used, unless extreme exertion is taking place, just like people with healthy lungs.

Quite simply, this technique teaches very natural breathing. It is relatively stress free. And even when the lungs are really badly affected by COPD, it can provide some degree of relief for the patient, something my patients are usually very appreciative of.

Exhalation – the driving force of breathing for the COPD lungs

Over the years of working with COPD patients I have found that, whilst I had been taught to place an emphasis on training people to actively breathe air into their lungs, it appeared to cause them considerable stress. Most patients had already learned to suck the air in hard, or had been taught previously to do so. I found that active inhalation training did not seem to relax patients very much. In fact, it seemed to have the exact opposite effect, making them appear very stressed, tight and anxious.

I learned to adjust my emphasis from active inhalation to active exhalation from an open chest. This seemed to work so I focused on two existing breathing techniques: pursed-lip breathing and paced breathing. I use the pursed-lip breathing technique as it has been used in yoga for centuries and modern physiotherapy worldwide. I also practised a range of paced breathing techniques similar to those that are used to promote healthy breathing and found a pace that seemed to work very effectively for patients with COPD.

Pursed-lip breathing

Breathing out through pursed lips can act to help regulate the speed and extent of exhalation. Think of letting air escape from your mouth as if you are trying to flicker the flame of a candle in front of you rather than huff and blow the candle out. This technique is used in many exercise routines, from yoga to weight-lifting to Pilates and in COPD rehab programmes, and is the only one of the four traditional COPD breathing techniques that I find useful with almost every patient. It is especially useful during the more advanced parts of the Brice Method, when patients are progressing to becoming more physically active.

A slow and controlled exhalation allows time for the oxygen in the deep alveoli to diffuse across into the bloodstream. If you blow out too hard or too quickly, the air that is in your lungs gets expelled before the oxygen has had time to move across to the blood.

Pursed-lip breathing also acts to prime the lungs effectively. I want you to picture in your mind a plastic bag that is held open with lots of air inside. If you keep the mouth of the bag wide open and push the sides of this bag inwards, all the air will rush out in a quick huff. The airflow is unrestricted and the bag collapses pretty much completely, all at once. When I watch my patients breathe out through a fully open mouth, this is how deflated their lungs and their chest look to me.

In contrast, once again picture the fully open bag of air. This time I want you to think about closing up the mouth of the plastic bag so there is only a small gap for air to pass out. Pushing the sides of the bag will cause a build-up of pressure, with a controlled flow of air going out. Picture the bag expanding out as the air is pushed out steadily. Think how a similar airflow out of the mouth would help increase the pressure in the exhaling lungs.

A good (but somewhat extreme) example of how this pursed-lip breathing can help with physical activity is looking at how Olympic weight-lifters expel the air with a hiss when they are lifting a heavy weight. Imagine how weak the lifter would be if he/she allowed air to escape too quickly through a fully open mouth. He/she would have all the strength of a floppy lettuce leaf, and there would be a lot of deflated weight-lifters lying prostrate on the floor!

At rest, exhaling slowly and gently can mimic the feeling of sighing. When we sigh, it has a very relaxing and calming effect on the body. Contrast this to when a patient is struggling to get enough air in, and the feeling of panic that this creates, and you can see why focusing on the exhalation is so important.

When the lungs have been emptied, the body automatically draws air in, partly by the natural action of the diaphragm drawing down into the space above the gut and partly due to the recoil of the elastic membranes of the bronchioles and alveolar ducts.

Adding pressure to the exhaled air has another beneficial effect for the body. If the exhaled air is at a relatively low pressure in the lungs, the pressure of gases is rather like what you might find at high altitude. Mountaineers take oxygen with them as they climb to combat the rarefied air. The air pressure is lower than that at sea level and oxygen is absorbed much less efficiently into the bloodstream. Exhaling through pursed lips increases the air pressure considerably, rather like the air pressure at sea level where oxygen is taken up more readily by the bloodstream.

Pacing and timing

The pace at which you breathe is the second key aspect of exhaled breath control that is generally most effective when used alongside the pursed-lip breathing you have just been told about. Paced breathing for COPD patients tends to be taught in a ratio of 2:4, that is, you should breathe in for a count of 2 and out for a count of 4. The idea is that you learn to slow your breathing rate down and allow a longer period of time for the oxygen to diffuse into your bloodstream from the alveoli over a count of 4.

This 2:4 breathing technique is used extensively for meditation, but when a COPD patient starts to be active, they have tended to find the 6 counts to be too long for their reduced capacity to manage. I worked alongside my patients to find the pacing that seemed to be most effective and it surprisingly matched the rhythm that front crawl swimmers use. This pacing time of '3:1' for the 'out:in' breath cycle was the one that patients appeared to find the most natural for them. Over time I have found this timing works especially well for walking or rhythmic cardiovascular type exercises, and is thus a great one to practise and adopt early on in training programmes.

As some patients count faster than others, especially if they are stressed out, I teach them all to do what I call 'parachute counting'. When a free-fall parachutist jumps out of a plane, instead of counting 'one', 'two' and so on, they count 'one thousand', 'two thousand' before pulling the cord to release the parachute. Adding the word 'thousand' to their count helps them to retain the single second spacing between the numbers counted. In doing so, they get enough space between them and the next person jumping out of the plane so that they do not get someone landing on top of their parachute.

Parachute counting

Before you try this breathing exercise, read it thoroughly and understand what you have to do. Only once you feel you understand what you need to do should you try the actual exercise that follows. This exercise should help expand your lungs automatically, drawing air into your lungs naturally.

To fully understand this breathing technique, you are required to count to yourself in 'parachute numbers'. As explained above, this means that each time you say 'one thousand', approximately one second will pass.

- Without first breathing in, gently exhale, through pursed lips, saying slowly to yourself: 'one thousand, two thousand, three thousand'.
- Inhale passively whilst slowly saying to yourself: 'one thousand'. (You will be surprised that your lungs draw air in without you having to work, as long as you don't slump!)
- Continue to breathe in this simple cycle. If you get the timing correct, each breath cycle will take you approximately 4 seconds and your breathing rate will be limited to 15 per minute, generally slower than would normally be the case for people suffering from COPD.

It is important that you do not suck air in deeply at the start of this exercise. You should have enough in your lungs to exhale for a 'three thousand' count. Inhaling at the start is likely to make you focus on inhalation rather than exhalation. Also, do not try to fully empty your lungs as this will add tension to the stretch receptors in your lungs and make you suck in hard for the next breath.

Sometimes patients find that if they do this exercise at complete rest they do not need much oxygen at all. You may find it takes a little longer than the 'one thousand' count for the lungs to draw air in again. My advice is not to push or rush the in-breath, at least until you start adding some of the more active exercises to the technique. The prime concern is to avoid sucking the air in actively as this will simply add stress to the situation.

Paced breathing

- Sit tall and comfortably.
- Without first breathing in, gently exhale, through pursed lips, counting: 'one thousand, two thousand, three thousand'.
- Inhale passively for a count of 'one thousand'.
- Repeat this cycle.

Advice

If you are finding it difficult to exhale slowly for the count of 'three thousand', then you are most likely forcing the air out too fast. It is easy to try and blow very hard so that almost all the air is expelled in the first 'one thousand'. By doing this you are stressing your respiratory system as you will have no air left in your lungs to take you to the full 'three thousand' count. It also means that you will have the air in your lungs for less time. This will limit the ability of your blood to take up the oxygen from the alveoli. It will also mean that you are highly likely to go into the '15% stress zones' that I explained in Chapter 2 (pages 33-4).

Inhalation muscle training

Inhalation muscle training may not be ideal for the COPD lung. In Chapter 2 of this book I mentioned the conventional advice on breathing techniques and highlighted the fact that the abdominal breath training focused on inhalation. I briefly covered the fact that focusing on inhalation may lead a person with COPD to have to work harder than they should need to in order to breathe. The three main reasons why I prefer not to emphasise inhalation muscle training for early stage COPD patients are as follows.

1. If your rib cage is already expanded by good posture, you are unlikely to need to strengthen your inhalation muscles to any real degree. That is, at least until you are exercising really hard. It is unlikely that many COPD patients will be able to, or expect to, work hard enough to have to train very strong inhalation muscles. If the body is positioned correctly, the diaphragm does not have to exert effort to push the belly down, plus the ribs do not have to be forced up against the tight chest muscles. In addition, the shoulder blades do not have to lift the weight of the head, as it is already balanced in its rightful place.

2. Inhalation can, and should, be a relatively passive and stress-free action. I believe it is wrong to teach patients to breathe in very hard as it is much more likely to be stress inducing and will do little for reducing anxiety or breathlessness. Inhaling too strongly increases the likelihood of the lung over-expanding into the 15% stress zone.

3. I believe that active inhalation training is not good for COPD patients because it promotes the same modified breathing pattern that smokers use when they take a drag on a cigarette. Over many years of practice, smokers learn a different way of breathing than the rest of us. They suck on their cigarette using mainly their neck muscles. This acts to engage the accessory muscles at the front of the neck, inducing the tight upper crossed breathing that many COPD patients demonstrate, and may even be due to the new movement patterns learnt when drawing in smoke. I teach these patients how to breathe in a relaxed, not a

tense, fashion. All you need to do is imitate the drawing in of smoke from a cigarette and you feel that the air is being sucked into the back of your throat, by neck muscles. If you are a non-smoker, think about sucking on a straw. Have you ever had a very thick milkshake and got tired neck and face muscles when it was too thick to suck? That can be the extreme feeling you get if you have COPD and are struggling to get air into your lungs.

Nasal breathing

Many of the new patients that I speak to have been told always to breathe in through their nose. They sit with their mouths clamped shut, sometimes sniffing air noisily in through their nostrils, even if they have nasal congestion, an exacerbation of breathlessness, or even when they are trying to be physically active.

There are pros and cons to teaching nasal breathing to COPD patients. When I was taught how to show COPD patients to breathe there was great emphasis on the benefits of nasal breathing. I worked with this technique, prompted by the evidence of research demonstrating everything from the fact that the hair in the nose filters the air, the folds in the soft palate warm the air up, and the cells in the nasal cavity release minute amounts of nitric oxide to act as an antiseptic to the cell linings of the lungs.

Most breathing programmes nowadays emphasise the benefits of nasal breathing and seem by default to have been used as the go-to technique for COPD patients. There are even those who advocate nasal breathing to extreme levels, recommending that you should nose-breathe when you run. The idea here is it will help you run faster.

I have found that whilst this breathing pattern is very useful for people with healthy lungs, patients with COPD seem to benefit more from having a more open airway, without the restriction of having to breathe through small nasal passages. This is especially the case when they have started to become active and their requirement for unrestricted air into their lungs seems more important than its warmth or the presence of minute molecules of nitric oxide, etc.

I have good reason to decry the overuse of nasal-only training, this time, from my experience as an athlete. If I ever saw an athlete racing an endurance race on the track and they were breathing solely through their nose with their mouth clamped shut, I would either show you someone who would be in great pain within three minutes, or alternatively, someone who was destined to come last. The simple fact of the matter is that when the body has an oxygen demand greater than it is currently receiving, you need to get the air in quickly, effectively, and in as stress-free a way as possible. This is exactly how I train my patients to breathe. That is, at least until they can use their lungs in a more normal, healthy pattern without stress. The reality of the situation is that a COPD patient is challenging their lungs to almost the same extent as a runner, so it makes sense to me to get as much air into the lungs as the body needs.

Another reason I try to avoid nasal-only breathing techniques for COPD patients is that recent research has demonstrated how strong nasal breathing recruits the accessory muscles of the neck. These are the weak and inefficient muscles that merely act to lift the top two ribs. Finally, I strongly feel that COPD patients should start by avoiding nasal-only inhalation, especially when they are being physically active, because it acts by restricting the refill rate of the lungs, creating a relative pressure vacuum that forces the patient to rely entirely on muscular effort to inhale. Sniffing air in hard can thus induce stress and agitation, exactly what I try to tell my patients to avoid at all costs.

Exercise to demonstrate nasal breathing issues for COPD patients

Compare these two simple exercises.

Closed-mouth inhalation

- Put one hand around the front of your neck, gently touching your skin.
- Empty your lungs as fully as you can, and then …
- with your mouth closed shut, suck air into your lungs as quickly and as deeply as you can.

Not only will you notice that it takes several seconds to fully expand your lungs, you will probably feel how strongly it makes the sinewy neck muscles tighten up as they activate; you are also likely to find it quite noisy in your head, and I doubt that you will find it truly comfortable, as it is quite hard to suck enough air in.

Now try the next exercise.

Open-mouth inhalation

- Put one hand around the front of your neck, gently touching your skin.
- Empty your lungs as fully as you can, and then ...
- breathe in equally through your mouth and the nose.

You will immediately see what I mean. There is less tension stress in the neck and the air travels in much more easily, without as much need to rely on the work of the neck muscles.

I fail to see why we would promote 'nasal-only' breathing as a good breathing technique for COPD patients who are just starting to learn how to overcome their dysfunctional breathing patterns. Personally, I recommend this technique only for those patients who get close to full use of their lungs. Healthy individuals can really benefit from nasal-only breathing, and this is well documented.

I maintain that, if the rib cage is expanded and lifted and the lungs are open, inhalation should be a relatively passive, natural and stress-free action.

Abdominal breathing

The last of the four breathing techniques that are currently used to help COPD patients overcome breathlessness is abdominal breathing. Personally, I feel that abdominal breathing comes about as an automatic result of good posture, rather than being an exercise to be learned in its own right.

This technique has already been discussed in Chapter 2 (see Figure 2.1). Pilates and yoga have similar techniques where you focus on expanding your ribs outwards. These aim to train you to actively engage and strengthen your diaphragm.

It is not that I disagree with the fact that working the diaphragm is important, it is simply that I find that COPD patients are better focusing on posture first, and the diaphragm will automatically engage as a result of having space to work in.

Unfortunately, whilst patients should always be told to first sit tall, this is not always the case. In my experience, rarely is there any real emphasis placed upon proper posture *before* undertaking breathing training. Failure to recognise the importance of posture means that many patients move straight to the breathing exercises and are more likely be under greater pressure than they would otherwise have to be.

Are you ready to progress?

Learning how to breathe in, without having to actively suck the air in, is a skill that will help you to master the art of relaxed natural breathing. This, combined with an upright controlled posture, can reduce the stress and tension in the body, and even mitigate feelings of anxiety that come with breathlessness.

Once you feel that you have can sit up tall and control your breathing so that you are not gasping or activley sucking the air in, you should think about moving on to Chapter 6 of the Brice Method. If, however, you still feel that you are very breathless and sucking the air in, do not worry. It may be that you need to practise the postural adjustments further and allow your body adequate time to change. Your current posture is likely to have taken years, if not decades, to form, and it won't always be able to change immediately.

Chapter 6

Upper body mobilisation and breathing

Once you have mastered the steps of awareness, posture and the effective breathing technique from the previous chapters, the next step is to learn how to sequence upper body movements in with your breathing. It is all very well to breathe comfortably when you are sitting or standing still and not expending any physical energy. Being physically active is another ball game altogether if you have COPD.

In this chapter, I start off by showing you how very simple arm movements enhance the postural changes you have already made, and how they can minimise the need to actively suck air in, even during gentle types of physical activity.

There are six upper body exercises included in this chapter. They aim to teach you how the muscles in your upper body can help you control your lungs to expand and draw air in passively, and how the direct opposite movement of the arms will allow your lungs to contract naturally, gently forcing the air out again. Combining these exercises with your paced breathing techniques may give you further insight into how easy, natural and stress-free breathing can be using the Brice Method.

Earlier on in this book I provided some health warnings and explained the difference between discomfort, good pain and bad pain. If you have jumped ahead to these exercises in this chapter, please read the Introduction now. However, in addition there are a couple of specific tips I would like to reiterate for you for the exercises that follow.

Choosing whether to sit or stand

The first five exercises can be done either seated or standing and, the final one can only be done standing. It is entirely up to you how you do them. If you are unsteady on your feet, I would advise you start them in the seated position, as there is less for you to think about, and they are no less effective. If you are quite fit and well and find the exercises easy, you can probably do them standing up, as they are likely to be easier to fit into your active daily lifestyle.

Advice to follow if seated

If you choose to do these exercises seated, you are best to use a firm chair, such as a dining chair or office chair. It should have an upright back and be stable, so you don't slump. If you do not have a firm, upright chair, try perching on the front of the seat you have and keep your body erect with your shoulder blades drawn back and downwards.

Otherwise, sit with your bottom as far back in the seat as possible, so that your body weight is on the top of your hamstrings, below your buttocks. This will stabilise your pelvis, lengthen your back and allow for better posture higher up your back and neck. Do not sit on your tailbone or feel too much pressure on the top of your buttocks, as this will cause you to slump.

Advice to follow if standing

If you prefer to do these exercises standing, you will need to remember to keep your knees slightly bent at all times. Not like a chimpanzee, but with a slight bend at the knee of, say, 3 or 4 degrees. Keeping your knees bent has the effect of making your hips stable, and stops your pelvis from tilting forwards, spilling your intestines forwards, and helps stop you from putting strain on both your abdominals and your lower back.

Keep your head looking straight forwards and ensure that your belly is not lolling forwards and causing your pelvis to tilt forwards excessively.

Dumb waiter exercise

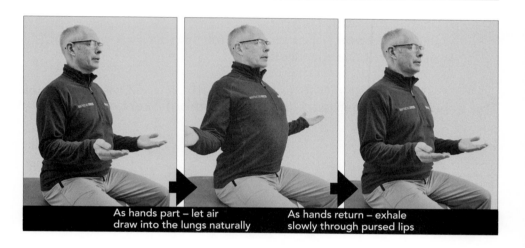

As hands part – let air draw into the lungs naturally

As hands return – exhale slowly through pursed lips

Figure 6.1 *The dumb waiter exercise*

- Sit or stand tall with your elbows tucked in to the side of your waist.
- Hold your hands in front of you with elbows bent and palms facing up.
- Keep your elbows touching the sides of your waist at all times.
- Spread your hands apart as far as you feel comfortable.
- Squeeze your shoulder blades together and downwards.
- Your chest will expand, and your lungs will automatically want to draw in air.
- Allow your lungs to fill naturally and don't suck the air in.
- Relax your hands and bring them back to the starting position, exhaling slowly through pursed lips.

71

Repeat the above sequence four times, inhaling for a 'parachute count' of 'one thousand', and exhaling for 'one thousand, two thousand, three thousand' (see Chapter 5 for more details of exhalation exercises).

Fine-tuning the dumb waiter exercise

- If you experience pain in the top of your shoulder, try repeating it with your palms facing together rather than upwards. If you still get pain, try once more with your palms facing down. This can change the way the bicep ligaments pull on your shoulder joints.
- As you get more used to the exercise you will find your chest and ribcage will expand more freely as your ribs loosen up.

The hand behind the head (Eric Morecambe) exercise

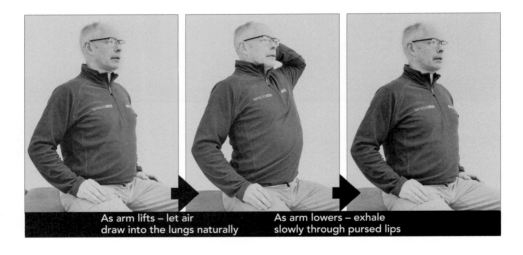

As arm lifts – let air draw into the lungs naturally

As arm lowers – exhale slowly through pursed lips

Figure 6.2: *The hand behind the head (Eric Morecambe) exercise*

- Sit or stand tall with your hands relaxed lying gently on the upper part of your thighs.
- Draw your shoulder blades back and down.

- Sit or stand tall with your eyes looking ahead.
- Put one hand behind your head with the elbow held high and out wide.
- Raising your arm will lift and open that side of your chest.
- The lung on that side will want to draw air in automatically.
- Allow this lung to fill naturally, don't suck the air in.
- Bring your hand back down to the start position, exhaling slowly through pursed lips.

Repeat the above sequence four times, alternating your arms, inhaling for a 'parachute count' of 'one thousand', and exhaling for 'one thousand, two thousand, three thousand'.

Fine-tuning the hand behind the head exercise

- Don't drop your head forwards making it easier for your hand to reach behind it, as this defeats the object of the exercise and is a cheat.
- If raising your elbows high is very painful, it is best to try doing the upright row (see below, page 74) and dumb waiter exercises to loosen up the shoulder girdle first. You might then like to attempt this exercise when you feel more flexible in the shoulder.

Seated row exercise

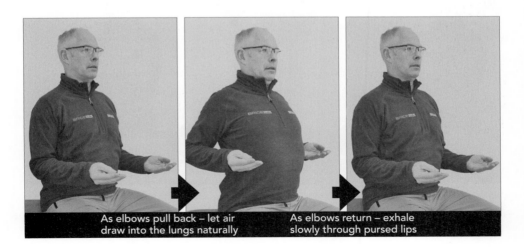

As elbows pull back – let air draw into the lungs naturally

As elbows return – exhale slowly through pursed lips

Figure 6.3: *The seated row (Fonzie) exercise*

- Sit or stand tall with your hands held in front of you and with your thumbs up.
- Pull your elbows backwards and together.
- Squeeze your shoulder blades together as your elbows draw back.
- Your rib cage will expand, drawing air into your lungs.
- Allow your lungs to fill naturally; don't suck the air in.
- Relax your hands and bring them back to the starting position, exhaling slowly through pursed lips.

Repeat the above four times, inhaling for a 'parachute count' of 'one thousand', and exhaling for 'one thousand, two thousand, three thousand'.

Fine-tuning the seated row exercise

- Don't drop your head forwards, as this defeats the object of the exercise.
- If you feel pain, don't pull your elbows back so far. You should gradually try to increase the range of motion over time, and you should feel your body loosen up.

The upright row (stirrup pump) exercise

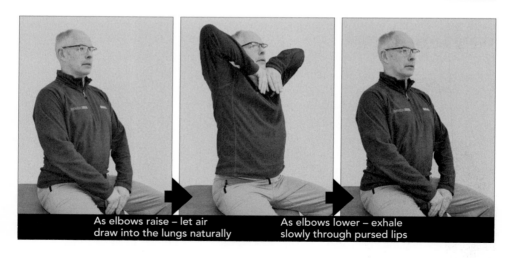

As elbows raise – let air draw into the lungs naturally

As elbows lower – exhale slowly through pursed lips

Figure 6.4: *The upright row (stirrup pump) exercise*

- Sit or stand tall, keeping your head held high, looking horizontally ahead.

- Grip hold of one thumb with the other hand.
- Slowly, draw your thumbs under your chin, pulling your elbows upwards and backwards.
- Finally squeeze your shoulder blades together.
- These actions all expand your chest and your lungs will want to draw air in.
- Allow your lungs to fill naturally, and don't suck the air in.
- Bring your hands back to the starting position, exhaling slowly through pursed lips.

Repeat the above four times, inhaling for a 'parachute count' of 'one thousand', and exhaling for a 'parachute count' of 'one thousand, two thousand, three thousand'.

Fine-tuning the upright row exercise

- If both shoulders are painful, ensure your shoulder blades are squeezed back and down, and re-try. It may be your shoulders are hunched forwards. If they still hurt, don't lift your elbows as high to start with and gradually increase the range of motion, as you feel capable.
- If only one of your shoulders is painful and squeezing your shoulder blades back and down does not help, try doing the exercise with only one arm at a time.

The shoulder lift exercise

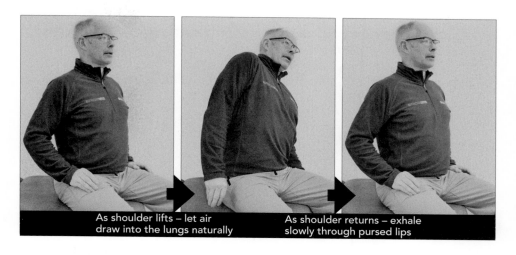

As shoulder lifts – let air draw into the lungs naturally

As shoulder returns – exhale slowly through pursed lips

Figure 6.5: *The shoulder lift exercise*

- Stand or sit tall with your eyes looking ahead.
- Have your hands on your hips or hanging at the sides of your body, shoulders drawn down.
- Raise the point of one shoulder near to the same height as your ear.
- This will expand the top part of your chest on that side of your body.
- Your chest will expand, drawing air into the lung on that side automatically.
- Allow this lung to fill naturally.
- Bring your shoulder back down to the starting position, exhaling slowly through pursed lips.

Repeat this sequence four times, alternating your shoulders, inhaling for a 'parachute count' of 'one thousand', and exhaling for 'one thousand, two thousand, three thousand'.

Fine-tuning the shoulder lift exercise

- If you feel pain or discomfort in your lower back, ensure that you are not slumping the opposite shoulder down rather than lifting the active shoulder up. This can pinch the nerves between the vertebrae. Ideally you should feel lifted and extended rather than compressed.

The wall press-ups exercise

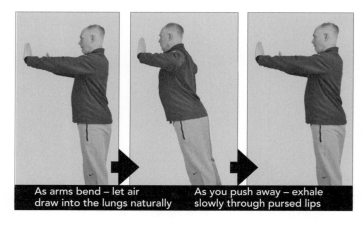

As arms bend – let air draw into the lungs naturally

As you push away – exhale slowly through pursed lips

Figure 6.6: *Wall press-ups*

- Stand facing towards a wall, with your feet an arm's-length from the wall.
- Place both hands on the wall in front, shoulder width apart, at chest height.
- Bend your arms slowly, letting your elbows draw apart.
- As you lean forwards, squeeze your shoulder blades together behind you.
- Your chest will expand, and your lungs will automatically draw in air.
- Allow your lungs to fill naturally and don't suck the air in.
- Exhale actively through pursed lips as you straighten out your arms to return to the starting position.

Repeat this up to 10 times, inhaling for a 'parachute count' of 'one thousand', and exhaling for 'one thousand, two thousand, three thousand'.

Fine-tuning the wall press-ups exercise

- If your wrists or hands are inflexible and cannot bend backwards enough to keep the palm of your hand on the wall, you can try using a clenched fist against the wall. If that is uncomfortable, the most forgiving way of doing this exercise is to stand in a doorway and put your palms on the doorframe at either side, with your fingers pointing inwards. This will enable you to do the exercise without having to bend your fingers back at 90 degrees and has the added benefit of directing your elbows up and outwards as you lean forwards.

How often should you do these exercises?

If I were to ask you to learn a short saying in another language, and for you to repeat it a week later, you would need to practise the saying daily, or risk getting it wrong. Obviously, the consequences of forgetting a random saying are minimal, but forgetting how to breathe and exercise well have massive potential implications for you. That means you need to do the exercises regularly!

I usually encourage my patients to do these exercises on a regular basis by being firm. I have found that only with repetition can you undo your old breathing habits. Often, we are trying to undo habits that will have formed over a considerable period of time.

You should aim to do:
- four of the upper body exercises (choose those you prefer)
- four repetitions of each exercise (wall press-ups, you can do 10)
- four times a day to help you remember them.

Do not try to do more repetitions as you will over-breathe and feel unwell.

As you do the arm exercises, you will most likely find that your joints will gradually start to feel less 'rusty'. It might take a couple of sessions, a couple of days or a couple of weeks for you to really feel the full benefit. I find that it helps enormously if you visualise your joints lubricating themselves as you move, especially at the start when movement feels a bit like a joint that has been taken out of the fridge. As your body starts to warm up and regain some of its natural range of motion you will be thankful that you put in the time and effort to do so. You are likely to be surprised at how wonderful it feels when your joints are looser and more relaxed. You should remember your body is designed to self-heal. It is simply amazing!

All five of these arm exercises are designed to be very simple and very gentle. They should not be hard work. The aim is first to re-learn how to sequence the breath along with movement, and secondly to realise that the correct movements will automatically allow your lungs to fill and empty without having to suck or blow too hard.

One thing you can remember as you practise, we humans are exactly like other members of the animal kingdom, and it is nature's way for the structure and function of the body to drive normal respiration. If only we had not invented the sofa, things might be a little better for our lungs.

The science behind the upper body exercises

If you want to understand in more depth what is happening to your body with these upper body exercises, you can read this section. If you feel you want to skip this section, you will not be any less able to complete the exercises effectively.

1. By sitting or standing tall, the postural benefits of expanding the rib cage are maximised.
2. The arm movements all pivot about the collarbones' (clavicles') attachment

to the sternum at the front of the chest, causing the shoulder blade to find its rightful place to the rear and lower down the rib cage than would normally happen.

3. The squeezing together of the shoulder blades as the elbows are drawn back in the dumb waiter, the Fonzie and the press-ups exercises, places further pressure on the rib cage to push forwards and expand, further expanding the lungs, drawing more air in. The opposite is the case as the arms and shoulder blades return forwards to their starting position and the air is expelled naturally. This sequencing of movement and breathing is a key skill that you will hopefully re-learn, with thoughtful and careful practice.

4. The raising of the shoulder blades as the elbows are drawn upwards in the Eric Morecambe, upright row and shoulder lift exercises, acts by drawing up the ribs as the shoulder blade is lifted. This expands the rib cage and opens the lungs in a different fashion from the first two exercises. This means that the exerciser does not exhale as he/she does the active part, but lets the air draw in as he/she lifts. The air is then expelled as the arms and shoulder blades return back down to their starting position and the rib cage lets air flow out of the gradually compressed lung.

5. Allowing air in through *both* the nose and the mouth during the various movements helps to reduce the air resistance as the air is drawn in. Doing this means that inhaled air resistance is reduced by a third, enabling the expanding lungs to do their work without having to rely as heavily on the muscles of inhalation, especially those that are normally overactive in nose-only breathing, such as the scalenes in the neck. By reducing the reliance on these small, weak muscles, you will feel the air travelling into your lungs naturally and without undue effort.

6. By exhaling through pursed lips, the flow of air slows down, and this allows the breathing rate to reduce. If the exhalation is executed evenly over the count of 'one thousand, two thousand, three thousand', there is less likelihood of the out breath being stressful. If all the air is pushed out in the first 'one thousand' of the count, the third 'one thousand' count will undoubtedly be hard work, as the exerciser will try to over-exhale.

7. By exhaling through pursed lips rather than an open mouth, there is a slight increase in the residual pressure inside the lungs, and this can help prime the lungs. Priming the lungs is where there is enough pressure inside them to push

the air into some of the collapsed alveoli, deeper within. This can have the effect of allowing air to travel deeper into the lungs. (There is one possible side effect from this, which is that air gets deeper into the lung than the areas where the mucus gathers, and it can make the exerciser want to cough more than usual.)

8. By using pursed-lip breathing and controlling the exhaled breath, it is possible to influence the intra-abdominal pressure which helps to engage the core muscles of the stomach and back to provide stronger, better coordinated movements.

All of the above techniques will be essential basic skills that can be related to more dynamic or more intensive types of activity as you progress and get fitter, and your breathing allows you to do more.

Are you ready to progress?

Your body is designed to breathe as you move. These upper body exercises impact directly upon your rib cage to help you control the amount of air that goes in and out of your lungs. This should result in a gentle and natural breath, and you should not feel uncomfortable or get breathless doing them.

Once you feel that you have gained the full benefit of coordinating these simple upper body movements along with your inhalation and exhalation, you should think about moving on to Chapter 7 of the Brice Method – Synchronising lower body movements with breathing.

If you do get breathless doing these exercises, or start feeling woozy or at all uncomfortable, don't try to move on. My advice is to go back and practise these upper body exercises a little more, listening to your body and mastering the techniques before your try to progress.

Chapter 7

Synchronising lower body movements and breathing

◊   Learning to move your lower body correctly

◊   High knee lift exercise

◊   Heel to bottom exercise

◊   Sit stand exercise

◊   How often should you do these exercises?

◊   The science behind the lower body exercises

◊   Are you ready to progress?

The movement of the muscles in the lower body may appear at first glance to have less impact on our breathing than that of the muscles of the upper body. As most of the muscles of the lower body do not directly attach to the rib cage, you would be excused for thinking that they do not have a significant influence over the size and shape of the lungs in the same way that the muscles of the upper body do that you worked on in the last chapter.

However, lower body movements place considerable indirect influence on the lungs through their action on the pelvis. As you no doubt know, the pelvis is the bony structure that is attached to the lower part of the vertebral column, and acts like a suspended platform for the upper body to work from, and the legs to attach to. The pelvis is attached to the rib cage by the muscles of the back and the abdomen, which work together to pressurise the contents of the abdominal cavity. This process not only helps the body to maintain an upright stance, but also keeps the gut in place.

I mentioned earlier in the book that the diaphragm sits between the chest cavity and the abdominal cavity. The relative pressure between the chest cavity and the abdominal cavity plays an important part in the effective working of the diaphragm. The synchronised contraction of the abdominal muscles and the back muscles, alongside the muscles of the lower limbs, results in changes in the intra-abdominal pressure. This force pushes the pelvic floor downwards and the diaphragm upwards. As the forces involved in lower leg contractions tend to be powerful, the reactive forces the abdominals and back muscles have to create are considerable. This is why it is important to learn how to correctly synchronise active lower body movements with breathing patterns.

Most of the patients I meet have been relatively inactive for a long time. That is relative to how physically active they used to be a few years previously. Some have not done anything that could be seen as physically challenging for years, even decades. Many of these patients seem to have lost all awareness of how their body used to work, forgetting the normal patterns of movement and breathing that they would have followed automatically in their youth. Those who have a history of being active playing sport will understand what I mean. Even after decades of not doing a sport, one can try to remember how it felt to run, jump, kick or squeeze one's legs. I use these types of memories to try and reinstate a patient's natural movement patterns, through engaging the more emotive parts of the brain first. Try it yourself now. Think of something active you used to do well in your younger days, and how your muscles used to feel when you did it. It may seem automatic to breathe at a certain time when doing that activity. If that does not work for you, don't worry, the following exercises may help you remember how to breathe and move your lower limbs.

It is very common for respiratory patients to be expected to be able to do the simple movements I will go through below without being reminded of how to do them well first. They usually get their breathing patterns and movement patterns mixed up, and whilst it is not the end of the world and they can often get by, they do not ever seem to reach the full potential that their body could achieve. Some even find that, without having the full explanation of what and how they should be doing it, they never overcome their inability to be actively mobile on their legs again. I find that taking the time to demonstrate the simple movements before going on to more complex ones really helps to ingrain good breathing and movement habits before the body is challenged physically with walking or cycling. Doing these simple mobility exercises helps my more inactive patients overcome their unsteadiness before moving on. Once again, the vast majority of patients I work with have graunching hips or knee joints and weak leg muscles. Taking a week or so to master these exercises will help make you less weak.

Learning to move your lower body correctly

Lifting one knee forwards in front of us is one of the first movements we use when we try to walk. This uses the hip flexor group of muscles that pull on the top of the thigh to lift the leg forwards and up. These hip flexors are attached to the inner aspect of the pelvic girdle and the lumbar vertebrae of the spine (see Figure 7.1).

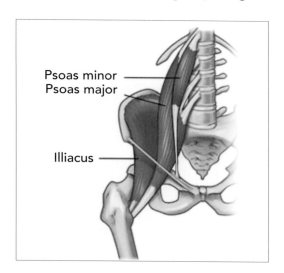

Figure 7.1: *The hip flexor group of muscles*

As the weight of the leg is being counterbalanced by the abdominals and back muscles to prevent the spine from being jerked forwards and causing pain in the back, teaching a person to contract the abdominals and back before the leg is lifted is extremely important. Contracting the abdominals and back is not enough to help the leg lift as high as it could, as the diaphragm also needs to work in synch with the other muscles, or the whole system fails. There are two errors that patients usually make in this movement.

1. The first mistake is for patients to hold their breath as they lift their leg. Holding their breath results in the diaphragm becoming an immovable object that prevents the abdominal mass from being squeezed upwards as the lungs reduce in size and limits the height that the knee can be lifted.

2. The second, and more common, mistake is for patients to breathe in as they lift their leg. This results in the diaphragm dropping downwards into the abdominal region, causing the abdominal muscles and back muscles to have no pressure to work against and they slacken off. This not only severely limits both the strength and the range of movement about the pelvis and hip, but also risks potential injury to the spine as the hip flexors work in isolation.

High knee lift exercise

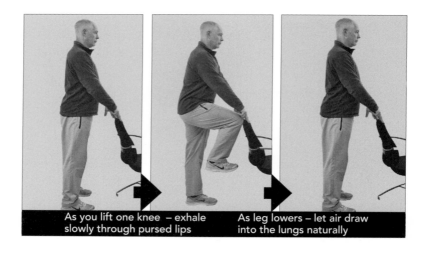

As you lift one knee – exhale slowly through pursed lips

As leg lowers – let air draw into the lungs naturally

Figure 7.2: *The high knee lift exercise*

- Stand tall with your shoulders back and your head looking straight ahead.
- Hold on to the back of a high chair or kitchen work surface, far enough away so you can lift a knee without banging it.
- Think about actively engaging your tummy muscles before you lift your leg.

84

- Exhale through pursed lips as you slowly lift one leg in front of you for a count of 'one thousand, two thousand, three thousand'.
- Let your leg lower and allow your lungs to fill naturally for a count of 'one thousand'.

Repeat the above sequence 10 times for each leg, alternating left and right, exhaling for a 'parachute count' of 'one thousand, two thousand, three thousand' and inhaling 'one thousand'. Make sure you only lift one leg at a time, or you will fall over! (Sorry, had to add that in.)

Fine-tuning the high knee lift exercise

- Keep your head held high so you can look straight ahead, with shoulders drawn back.
- Stand with soft knees, especially if you suffer from low back pain; bent knees will take the pressure off your spine.
- As you lift your knee, actively engage your tummy muscles to maintain pressure in the abdominal space, giving your diaphragm something to work against.

The heel to bottom exercise

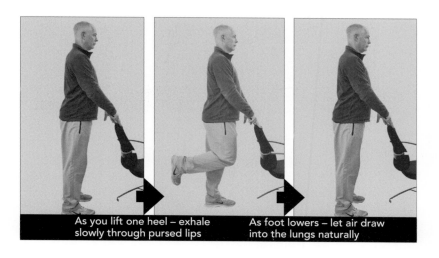

As you lift one heel – exhale slowly through pursed lips

As foot lowers – let air draw into the lungs naturally

Figure 7.3: *The heel to bottom exercise*

85

- Stand tall with your shoulders back and your head looking straight ahead.
- Hold on to the back of a high chair or kitchen work surface.
- Exhale through pursed lips as you slowly lift one heel behind you for a count of 'one thousand, two thousand, three thousand'.
- Don't jerk your leg up, or hold your leg up, as this can cause the hamstring to cramp.
- Let your foot lower and allow your lungs to fill naturally for a count of 'one thousand'.

Repeat the above sequence 10 times, alternating each leg, exhaling for a 'parachute count' of 'one thousand, two thousand, three thousand' and inhaling for 'one thousand'. Only lift one leg at a time!

Fine-tuning the heel to bottom exercise

- Stand with soft knees, especially if you have low back pain; bending your knees slightly can take the pressure off the spine.
- As you lift your heel, actively engage your tummy muscles to prevent your bottom from sliding backwards towards your heel as it comes up. This can also put additional pressure on your lower back.

The sit stand exercise

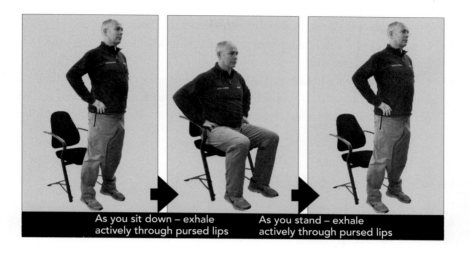

As you sit down – exhale actively through pursed lips

As you stand – exhale actively through pursed lips

Figure 7.4: *The sit stand exercise*

- Stand tall with your shoulders back and your head looking straight ahead.
- Let your calf muscles touch the front of the seat of the chair, so you know it is in place.
- Exhale through pursed lips and keep looking ahead as you slowly sit down.
- Count 'one thousand, two thousand, 'three thousand' as you sit, to control your descent.
- Pause whilst you sit, allowing your lungs to fill naturally for a count of 'one thousand'.
- Exhale through pursed lips and keep looking ahead as you slowly stand up again.
- Count 'one thousand, two thousand, three thousand' as you stand, to control your ascent.
- Pause whilst you stand, allowing your lungs to fill naturally for a count of 'one thousand'.

Repeat the above sequence up to 10 times, exhaling for a 'parachute count' of 'one thousand, two thousand, three thousand' and inhaling for 'one thousand'.

Fine-tuning the sit stand exercise

- Keep your head facing straight ahead, with shoulders drawn back.
- Stand with soft knees, especially if you have low back pain.
- If you feel unstable, make sure you keep your knees apart, tracking over the line of the second toe.
- Coordinating your breathing with this exercise may not be easy. Many people inhale as they stand. It won't hurt you to get the breathing mixed up, but do persevere, as the extra force you can get when you exhale will definitely benefit you in the long run.

How often should you do these exercises?

Just as with the previous set of upper body exercises, you need to do these lower body exercises regularly.

You should aim to:

- do only those exercises you feel comfortable doing
- continue with the arm exercises from the previous chapter
- do only 10 repetitions of each exercise
- do the new exercises four times a day, to help you remember them.

The science behind the lower body exercises

If you want to understand in more depth what is happening to your body with these lower body exercises, you can read this section. If you feel you want to skip this section, you will not be any less able to complete the exercises effectively.

1. The first two of these leg exercises are designed to be extremely simple and very gentle. They should not be hard work. Each of these exercises is designed not only to benefit your breathing pattern but also to strengthen muscles and loosen up the joints of the knee, hip and ankle. They will also help you work a little on balance, something that may be important for you as you start your exercising, especially if you have been inactive or bedridden for some time.

2. Both the high knee lifts and the heel to bottom are very useful to teach

you to lift your legs without hurting your back. By engaging your abdominal muscles actively as you lift your legs, you will support your lower torso, preventing your hip flexors that attach to the lower lumbar vertebrae from shunting the vertebrae forwards, and preventing possible nerve impingement. The exercise should help you if you want to use a bicycle to exercise. You often have to get your leg over a central bar to use a stationary bicycle, and these exercises help teach you to do that without getting completely breathless.

3. The sit stand exercise is a little more taxing, especially if you have severe mobility problems. However, the aim once again is to re-learn how to sequence your breathing along with leg and hip movements, allowing your lungs to automatically fill and empty without you having to suck or blow too hard. The intensity of the exercise will to some degree be dependent upon your body weight, so if you are overweight, you will need to take care not to overstrain your knees by going gung-ho at this. Remember you shouldn't go near the pain barrier. Strength will develop over time with regular and consistent repetition as the muscles store more energy, grow stronger and become better coordinated. If your legs shake a little at first, it is because the multitude of muscle fibres in your thighs and buttocks are not being sequenced effectively all together. Once your body wakes up, and re-learns the movement pattern, you should become stronger and more efficient.

4. Once you feel that you have gained the full benefit of opening your lungs and getting a steady relaxed breath coordinated with these lower body movements, you can then move on to the next stage: synchronising regular, rhythmic exercise with your breathing.

5. As you do these lower body exercises, you should find that your joints begin to feel less 'graunchy'. It might take you several sessions, a number of days or a couple of weeks. It will help if you picture your hip, knee and ankle joints lubricating themselves as you move, and, as with the upper body exercises, you should always remember that your body is designed to heal itself.

Are you ready to progress?

Your body is designed to breathe as you move. These lower body exercises indirectly affect the amount of air that goes in and out of your lungs. Practising these exercises should result in a gentle and natural breath, and you should not feel uncomfortable or get breathless doing them.

If you do get breathless doing these exercises, or start feeling woozy or at all uncomfortable, don't try to move on to the next sections yet. My advice is to go back and practise these movements a little more, listening to your body and mastering the techniques before your try to progress.

Once you feel that you have gained the full benefit of coordinating these simple lower body movements along with your inspiration and exhalation, you should think about moving on to Chapter 8 of the Brice Method (Breathing on the move), taking the time to repeat the Landmark Self-test on the next page (page 91), and comparing the result with your previous two scores (pages 13 and 56).

Landmark 3

Landmark 3 is a perfect time to re-visit the simple exercise test you have done twice before and see if you have improved enough to move on to the next stage of the Brice Method.

Self-test 3

Take a deep breath, and think about where you can feel the air inside your body. Draw on the picture of the torso below where you feel the air going in your body.

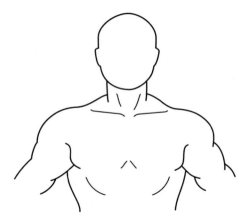

Once you have drawn the full extent of where you feel the air go into your chest, I would like you to note down how you would rate the quality of this breath on a scale of 1 to 10.

1	2	3	4	5	6	7	8	9	10
Poor				Average			Good		Fantastic

Check your scoring and compare this with the self-tests you did at Landmark 1 and Landmark 2. See if your score has improved.

Chapter 8

Breathing on the move

The most common mistake that I find my COPD patients make when they first start to walk or move more than a few yards without guidance, is that they forget to breathe.

It may sound silly that they have got to an age (in many cases a ripe old age) and forgotten the most basic life skill, especially when you consider the fact that a breath is pretty much the first thing they did when they were born, so they have been doing it all their lives.

Oddly enough, there is a good reason why this phenomenon occurs. The human body is quite capable of providing energy for muscular activity for a short period of time without using oxygen as the fuel. Thus, you can do a little bout of exercise without really having to use your lungs.

As some COPD patients have become extremely inactive, their bodies have learned how to rely on this alternative energy system to get them from A to B. With time, the cycle of deconditioning takes its toll and the body learns to use what is called the 'anaerobic' energy system rather than 'aerobic' (oxygen-based) energy system whenever stressed.

Here is a very simple explanation of the difference between aerobic and anaerobic energy systems.

- **Aerobic respiration**: The human muscular system that enables us to move is designed to work most effectively with oxygen as the energy source. This is called 'aerobic' respiration and the term translates as 'with oxygen'. By using oxygen as a fuel, the muscles can work pretty much until complete exhaustion, as long as the intensity of exercise is moderate enough not to over-tax the system. Distance running, cycling, hiking, rowing and exercise classes are all forms of aerobic exercise.

- **Anaerobic respiration**: Translated, 'anaerobic' means 'without oxygen'. Whilst the muscular system needs oxygen to work at its most efficient, there are times when we humans have had to react and move quickly and powerfully, even more quickly than it takes the heart and lungs to get pumping oxygenated blood round the body. Imagine our ancestors in the jungle, seeing a tiger about to pounce. If they had to wait for their heart and lungs to pump sufficient oxygenated blood to the relevant muscles, they would not have survived. To get an immediate boost of powerful energy to get away from the tiger, the anaerobic energy system uses energy that has been stored in the muscles to be used in times of extreme need. Using this form of stored energy is less efficient when compared with burning oxygen and gives off more waste products. Not only that, the anaerobic energy system has a finite supply of energy, and when you are working hard, you may find that it will only last up to a maximum of 90 seconds before it runs dry. Exercising without oxygen is also not a clean process; it gives off a lot of waste products (such as lactic acid) that sit in the muscles rather than getting flushed away by the circulating blood. This means that anaerobic exercise can not only be more painful for the muscles than aerobic exercise, but the build-up of waste products acts like a poison to the body and will ultimately limit further physical activity.

It is interesting to note that the most sedentary COPD patients tend to do only tiny bursts of activity. In doing so, they generally use the energy stored in their muscles anaerobically. These individuals rarely do any type of exercise for long enough to utilise their aerobic system, and it is little wonder that this system becomes deconditioned.

The good news is that there is a simple technique that can be used to combat this double-edged sword of a problem. It is to breathe *before* you move!

I have found the simplest way to teach patients how to breathe before they move is to use a visualisation exercise.

Visualisation exercise

Sit quietly away from distractions, close your eyes and picture the following:
- You are driving a car and you can see a big hill approaching.
- As you reach the bottom of the hill, you don't accelerate up the hill, but you maintain the same amount of throttle as when you were on the flat.
- If you did this you would soon find your car starting to lose momentum, the engine would start to strain and eventually might cough and splutter a little before stalling.

This might be exactly how your body reacts when you walk up a hill or flight of stairs if you have forgotten to breathe. Including the coughing and spluttering and coming to a grinding halt!

Now, picture the following:
- You are coming to the same hill and you start to accelerate well before the hill starts and continue to do so when you climb the hill.
- The car sweeps up the hill with no issues, no strain and no struggle.

This is what should happen to your body if you start to breathe a little harder before you come to a hill or flight of stairs.

If you practise, you can learn how to prepare your body for exercise well in advance and pre-oxygenate your blood, giving your body momentum where it used to have inertia.

How to pace your breathing

There are a number of breathing techniques designed to control the pace at which you breathe. Most have been developed not specifically for COPD patients but have been adapted slightly from those designed for healthy individuals. Most involve focusing on a long, deep inhalation, and long exhalation. The most common one used is to breathe in for a count of 4 and out for a count of 4. Having tried this with patients before I started focusing on correcting postural imbalances, sucking air in actively was the *only* way of getting air into their compressed lungs. However, I found that when my patients adopted an upright posture, their lungs were already quite open, and being full of air they only had to focus on a slow and controlled exhalation.

As described in earlier chapters, the pacing that my patients found the most natural was to say to themselves the words 'one thousand, two thousand, three thousand' as they breathed out and 'one thousand' as they breathed in. (By counting this way each breath takes approximately 4 seconds in total, giving a respiration rate of 15 breaths per minute. This pacing appears to be ideal for gentle exercise.)

This 3000:1000 ('parachute') pacing is easily coordinated with leg and arm movements, such as steps, pedals or strokes or any other rhythmic movement. I have used this as the starting point for working with patients, and whilst it does not have to be strictly adhered to, I have found that the simple 3:1 ratio works really well.

Exercises for paced rhythmic breathing

Choose whichever of these exercises suits you best:
- walking on the spot
- seated side punches.

If you can stand and move your legs comfortably and safely, try walking on the spot. If your legs are weak and unsteady or you have back, or joint, problems, try the seated side punches.

Walking on the spot exercise

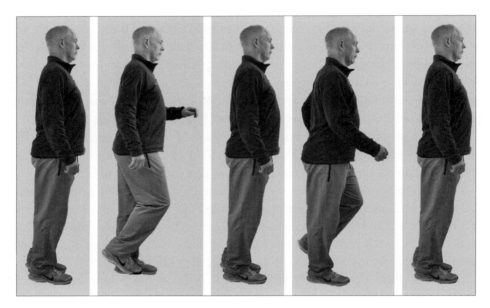

Figure 8.1: *Walking on the spot*

- Stand up tall with your shoulders back and your hands hanging loosely to the side of your hips (don't slouch).
- Start counting and controlling your breathing, counting to yourself 'one thousand, two thousand, three thousand' as you breathe out and 'one thousand' as you breathe in.
- After you have done three cycles of breathing, start adding leg movements to each count. This means you will be walking with three steps being timed with your **out** breath, and one step sequenced with your **in** breath.
- Repeat the cycle above, walking for between 10 and 20 cycles and then stand still. After you have stopped, you should continue to breathe in the 3000:1000 ratio as it is very common to return to the old habit of stopping activity and reverting back to gasping breaths for recovery.

Punching side to side exercise

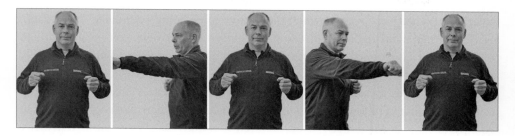

Figure 8.2: *Punching side-to-side*

- Perch on the front of a chair, sitting up tall with your shoulders and elbows back and hands in a fist to the side of your body. (Don't slouch.)
- Start counting and controlling your breathing counting to yourself 'one thousand, two thousand, three thousand' as you breathe out and counting 'one thousand' as you breathe in.
- After you have done three cycles of breathing, start punching across your body at approximately shoulder level, rotating your body about the erect spine, one arm movement to each count. This means you will be moving with three punches being sequenced with your **out** breath, and one punch sequenced with your **in** breath.
- Try punching for between 10 and 20 cycles and then stop. After you have stopped, you should continue to breathe in the 3000:1000 ratio, as it is very common for patients to have got into the old habit of stopping activity and reverting back to gasping breaths for recovery. Going back to your old habits could cause your breathing to become more distressing.

With either the walking or the punching exercise it is important that you try not to push yourself too hard. If you have learned the breathing patterns and breathing exercises to this point well enough, you should find these exercises surprisingly simple. You should also make sure you stop before you start feeling breathless. Getting very short of breath is counter-productive. I prefer my patients to feel in control. The stress and tension that come with being breathless mean you have lost control.

You should feel the muscles working gently and rhythmically, and if you can visualise your body being relaxed and calm, you are more likely to find that the movement feels good. After all, movement is a natural state for the human body. Nearly everybody feels good when they move after being stationary for a length of time. Enjoy that feeling and use it to reinforce your own self-awareness and improve your confidence in your body, so that you can move and not get terribly out of breath.

If you find it particularly hard to adopt this breathing pattern, I stress, the 3:1 pacing is not a strict rule to follow. You can for instance allow breath to take slightly longer to go in, so do not get concerned if every so often your body takes more air in, especially when you are first learning the technique. It is probable that you have developed quite ingrained breathing patterns, and it is therefore likely to take some time to override these habitual patterns.

You may find that you need to adopt a different breathing pattern of 4000 out:2000 in. Whichever pattern helps you to breathe *without* any feelings of stress and tension, especially in the neck and upper chest, will be good to start with.

Building up to doing true aerobic exercise

Continuous exercise that elevates the heart and breathing rate is called 'cardiovascular exercise', and as it is a bit of a mouthful, you will often find it commonly shortened to 'CV exercise'. If you do find yourself talking to a fitness instructor, you will undoubtedly hear the term CV training.

To do cardiovascular exercise over a prolonged period of time takes a little while to build up to. I tend to start patients off with short periods of gentle rhythmic exercise with rest periods in between, so that their breathing returns to normal. If you find one of the exercises above easy to do, you can then start to try other forms of exercise. Once again, the emphasis is on avoiding getting out of breath.

When starting patients on CV exercise I find that I have two challenges, depending upon the person I have in front of me. There are those who are really reluctant to do much CV exercise, as they have struggled excessively in the past, and those who push themselves too hard. My advice is the same for both. Work to the point that you start to feel your breathing rate and depth are elevated, but try to stop before you get out of breath, Avoiding the onset of fear, panic, frustration and embarrassment of being breathless is key to ensuring you progress. Don't over-do it!

Developing your ability and improving your confidence

Starting off slowly and gently for short periods of time and gradually building up the length of time you do is key. Don't be tempted to try and work too fast or too hard, too soon. All this will do is increase the likelihood of your getting out of breath faster.

I frequently start my patients off with four or five short bouts of 30 seconds to 1 minute of exercise with rest periods in between. The objective is to get the breathing pace correct, and to get them used to the idea that they can exercise and not be breathless. They are usually quite surprised when their breathing is comfortable and not challenging.

Within a couple of workout sessions, patients have usually built up to doing bouts of at least 2–3 minutes, again with short rest periods in between. Usually they will do several exercises in this fashion within one workout with other strength or mobility exercises.

Gradually, as the body acclimatises to the idea of moving, joints will start to feel as if they are warming up and becoming more mobile, the blood flows more readily, transporting oxygen, nutrients and waste around the body, and the breathing pattern often stabilises quite naturally. I am always amazed at how patients who have struggled to breathe at rest can actually manage to breathe with relative ease when they are getting used to being active again.

Once you start to feel the benefit of the naturally induced increase in respiration that accompanies exercise, you will start to take control over how much exercise you might be able to do. Do not be concerned if you are only able to increase this slowly. The speed of your progress is often related to the severity of your condition, and there is no magic formula. It is merely the consistency of your approach and your focus on getting the techniques correct that will help you progress as fast as your body will allow.

In my clinic, once a person has mastered the breathing sequence and does not show the signs of even mild breathlessness and moderate discomfort with their breathing for a couple of sessions in the gym, I will often let them decide how long they can keep up the exercise before they have to stop. Strangely, more often than not these patients will surprise themselves, and sometimes they will even surprise me. They will often work longer than they would have dared to dream possible a couple of weeks previously.

Choosing what rhythmic exercise to do

Your choice of exercise will depend ultimately on what other health conditions you may have, as well as the degree of restriction you have with your breathing.

I am fortunate enough to work in a commercial gym and I have access to a wide range of equipment that makes exercise safe and easy. Figure 8.3 gives a breakdown of the machine choices that I work with to build up stamina and train the cardiovascular system. If you have, or can get, access to such a facility, the various benefits to your cardiovascular system from the different exercise machines are shown in the chart.

	Intensity range 1 = Easy 10 = Hard	Postural support for COPD	Upper limb issues – shoulders/elbow etc	Lower limb issues – hip/knees/ankles/feet	Back problems
Recline bike	1 to 4	Excellent	Excellent	Excellent	Excellent
Arm bike	2 to 5	Good	Average	Excellent	Good
Uprightbike	1 to 5	Poor	Average	Good	Good
Treadmill walking	2 to 9	Good	Good	Average	Good
Cross trainer	3 to 7	Poor	Average	Poor	Average
Swimming	1 to 8	Good	Average	Good	Good
Rower	4 to 10	Average	Average	Poor	Average
Stepping machine	5 to 8	Poor	Average	Poor	Poor

Figure 8.3: *Cardiovascular exercise machine choice*

Listed below are my four preferred CV exercise options for those with COPD, along with my rationale for choosing them in this order.

Recline bike

A stationary recline bike is generally the CV exercise that I recommend most for patients with COPD to start with.

A recline bike allows you to sit down so you can exercise without all your body weight on your legs, unlike walking or other standing exercise. The back rest adequately supports your back, so it is great if you have a painful back or poor abdominal strength. The support from the back rest, and the fact that most have handles beside the seat, enables you to sit upright. You will find that if you do not use the handles in front of you (as if you are steering a normal bicycle), you can draw your elbows back behind you, and this will serve to further elongate your spine, opening up your chest cavity, with the ribs flaring out, and your sternum being lifted off your abdomen. Often you can immediately feel your breathing being driven by your diaphragm, and the emphasis being taken off the muscles in your neck and shoulders.

There are some patients whom a recline exercise bike does not suit. This does not always mean that a person will never be able to use this machine; merely that they need to do a little work to get their body ready to cycle. Having hip and knee joint pain (replacement joints are very common nowadays), plus very severe back pain, are the most common reasons that I do not recommend the recline bike to patients. With back pain, you may find you are unable to lift your knee to get your leg over the central part of the bike to sit down. Often if you practise the 'high knee lift' exercise from Chapter 7 (page 84), you can learn how to get your leg over. The limitation that some patients find with knee or hip joint replacements, or pain, may mean that they cannot get their leg to do a full cycle of the pedals. If this is the case for you, you might try to gradually build up the range of motion of your legs, or change the way you cycle. Sometimes people who can't complete a full cycle are not bending their ankle joint, making the knee and hip do all the work. By toe-ing (pushing the toe as you extend your leg away from your body, and pulling the toe back as your foot is pulled forward on the circular motion) will take up some of the effort and make it possible to pedal effectively and without discomfort or pain.

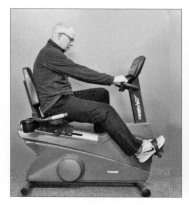 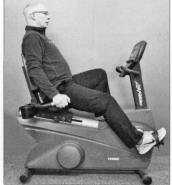

Figure 8.4: *Recline bike – bad versus good (straight, supported back) posture*

Arm bike

The arm bicycle, or 'arm ergometer' as it is sometimes known, is my second favourite CV machine to be used by patients with COPD. Those patients with leg or hip problems may not be able to do much exercise on their lower limbs, and this exercise is a great alternative. It can also be done seated, so body weight or deconditioned leg muscles are less of an issue.

As the name suggests, you can use an arm bike to work the upper body in a rhythmic fashion. You need to be sitting tall essentially, perching on the chair you are working from. Perching on the chair prevents you from sitting on it like a sofa, and elongates the spine, making each vertebra engage in almost every exercise, this one included. When you first start using the arm bike you will find that you tend to emphasise the use of your arms in isolation without trying to use the muscles of your back and waist.

You should sit tall, with your chest high, and your head up to ensure your body is not slumped. Your lungs will then be as open as can be before you start to pedal with your arms. When you do start to pedal you should sit leaning forwards slightly to engage your abdominal muscles and back muscles. Once you have got momentum in your arm movements, you should start to roll your shoulders, keeping your pelvis still on the seat. Rotating your shoulders so that your rib cage rotates slightly about the axis of your spine engages all of the postural muscles of your abdomen, back and chest, as well as all of the muscles that cause your spine to lengthen. This gives your body a more powerful shape to work from, and is the position you will see the sailors on the round-the-world sailing ships use to winch the main sails up.

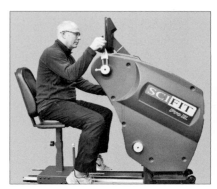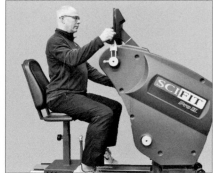

Figure 8.5: *Arm bike – bad versus good (straight back, open chest) posture*

Upright bike

Due to the fact that the seats on upright bikes are a little uncomfortable for the average unfit person, and because there is no back support, I have found that the upright bike is less ideal for COPD patients than the recline bike. The lack of a back rest means that you will tend to lean forwards, usually in a hunched position, which is more likely to collapse your lungs as your ribs are forced down on to the contents of your abdomen.

If you can maintain an upright posture, or if you can keep your spine relatively straight and do not feel too precarious, the upright bike can still be a good exercise to help develop your CV fitness. As the saddle supports you, you will find that your legs do not have to take 100% of your body weight and there is not the impact on the body that you can get from walking. In a similar fashion to the recline bike, the range of motion you need to complete the revolutions of the pedals may mean that those with replacement, or injured, knees and hips can be limited at first with their cycling. Saying that, it is rare that patients do not get to complete a full revolution comfortably after a few attempts. This may mean you have to persevere at first and keep trying, as well as doing the lower limb exercises like heel to bottom (page 85) in Chapter 7.

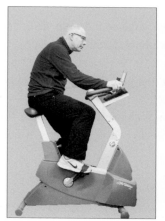 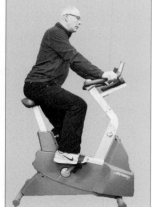

Figure 8.6: U*pright bike – bad versus good (straight back, open chest) posture*

Treadmill

To many of my patients the idea of walking on a treadmill seems a little daunting at first. Some have done challenging treadmill tests in hospital to monitor their heart's response to exercise, a test which at the best of times can be quite uncomfortable. Others will have seen the comedy of errors clips that are shown on the TV or on the Internet, and be rather worried they might 'come a cropper'.

There are several benefits in using a treadmill over walking outside. The first benefit is that if you get tired you can stop and don't have to walk back. This can be very useful if you do not have any idea of how far you can comfortably walk, especially if you are susceptible to exacerbations or panic attacks. Another benefit is that with correct training you can maintain a very good posture by holding on to the handles.

There are some simple tips as to how you should use a treadmill:

- Firstly, you should always try to stand tall, and not allow yourself to hunch forwards.
- You shouldn't grip the handles too tightly either, as doing this will put additional stress on the muscles of your shoulders and neck. Remember the amount of stress your neck muscles are under when your head is leaning forwards and you are looking down. (See Figure 3.2 in Chapter 3.)
- Thinking of this weight being like a yoke round your neck as you walk will certainly make you want to stay upright and not hunch over.

With a treadmill, it is probably obvious that you should start slowly and get into a rhythm.

One difficulty of using a treadmill is you do have to support your full bodyweight, something that you may find difficult if you have joint problems or poor balance.

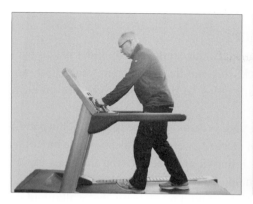 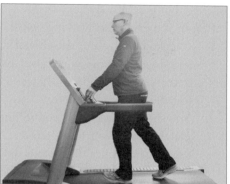

Figure 8.7: *Treadmill – bad versus good (straight back, open chest) posture*

I have found that other cardiovascular exercise machines are usually less effective for new COPD patients, either due to the simple fact that they are too demanding in terms of intensity, or they are more likely to need considerable strength to use them correctly.

At the end of the day, the single most natural form of cardiovascular exercise is walking. Walking may be quite challenging if you are just learning the breathing techniques, but the breathing pattern is the same 3000:1000 ratio, and this technique is explained in the next section.

Mastering walking and breathing

Very often I find that patients with COPD who have not been shown how to breathe properly when they are being active are in a hurry to get things over and done with to avoid having to tax their lungs unduly.

Walking is the most common activity that COPD patients are likely to avoid. I put this down, in part, to the fact that they will have learned to rely almost entirely on their anaerobic system to complete a task. This means that these patients will rush ahead and feel completely pooped before they have got more than a few yards. Doing this would not only break your confidence and cause you concern, but you can also get very frustrated, embarrassed or angry. Avoiding this can take a little practice, but is relatively easy to do.

Before you even start walking you should:

1. Check your posture. You should stand tall squeezing your shoulder blades back and down towards your lower back; this can help you open your chest, and make you think about what you are going to do and how you are going to breathe before you move.
2. You should think about controlling your breathing in a set pattern. This pattern matches the breath to the number of steps. As before in this book, the breathing sequence matches the 3 steps out, 1 step in approach. Using the steps as you breathe is a fantastic way of sequencing your breathing with your walking.
3. Make sure you don't take short steps. I jest with my patients that walking like a Geisha, or trotting along as if you have your trousers round your ankles, makes you take quick breaths, which is not very relaxing. Longer, slower strides are better for you as your breathing is less likely to be frantic.

Once you have practised walking like this for a while, you will probably find that you gradually start to relax a little as you walk. If you have become fearful of getting out of breath through walking, or if you get embarrassed or frustrated when not being able to do things you consider should be really easy, you may find it will take a little time before you can truly relax.

You should start with slow gentle strides, exhaling and counting to three, and letting the air flow back in naturally and not sucking for one step.

As you practise the three steps out/one step in walking pattern, you will eventually become more confident and are likely to start thinking about tackling more intensive challenges, such as walking upstairs, or even up hills.

When approaching stairs or hills, I ask patients to prepare themselves by starting to control their breathing a good few strides before they start climbing. They can do this by starting to breathe using the 3:1 exhalation to inhalation stride pattern.

This is rather like the visualisation exercise I explained earlier in this chapter. Imagine you are driving a car up to a hill and you start accelerating before you reach the hill. If you stand tall with your chest open, adopt the 3:1 ratio and slightly increase the depth of your breathing, you are less likely to cough and splutter up the hill or stairs.

With practice, many patients have told me that they do not have the same feeling of dread and panic as they used to when they have this challenge. Soon they feel that they do not have the same trepidation when they see stairs in a shop or when they visit someone's house with an upstairs toilet.

106

Eventually, the activities that you have practised in this chapter form habits you can replicate with whatever activity or form of exercise you choose to do.

The simple movement patterns that you practise time and time again will often re-awaken the body's natural breathing rhythm. I find it fascinating how so many of my early stage patients wander into the gym sessions saying that their breathing has been poor even when they have been resting, only to find that their breathing almost normalises once they start doing this gentle, rhythmic style of exercise. It is almost as if the body has stored the memory of how it should breathe normally, and keeps it secret until it is asked to do it well.

Are you ready to progress?

In this chapter you should have managed to practise and understand the need for a rhythmic, consistent pace to your breathing as you exercise. Practising these techniques will ultimately help you to get a more relaxed flow of air in and out of your lungs as you move. It is recommended that you maintain the practice described in the previous chapters and exercise four times a day, to help embed them as your new breathing habits.

If you feel that the 3:1 exhalation-to-inspiration ratio does not suit you, read through the chapter again and you will see that this is only a guideline; you may feel better with a slightly different ratio. Similarly, if you find the parachute counting 3000:1000 hard to master, do not worry. It is again just a guide that many people have found useful.

Once you feel that you have fully benefited from the exercises in this chapter, you should think about moving on to Chapter 9 - Increasing effort and developing strength.

Chapter 9
Increasing effort and developing strength

When starting this part of the Brice Method, you should by now have practised, if not mastered, simultaneously coordinating regular physical movements along with comfortable rhythmic breathing. In this chapter I will show you how you can build up to doing more vigorous types of exercise without getting really breathless. I can't promise that you will be able to do lots of high intensity exercise; that will depend on your overall state of fitness, and any other physical limitations and co-morbidities you may have. You should, however, be able to use these techniques to gradually build up your ability. The benefits of a steady and gradual increase in intensity are that you should not only become physically stronger, but you should also develop a great deal more confidence in your own abilities.

Before you start on the exercises in this chapter, I must caution you not to go gung ho with them. The aim is not to 'Get Fit Quick' in the traditional sense. You will need to take a little time to build up to a reasonable level of activity and load. I reiterate time and time again to my own patients that you don't have to work hard. I try to emphasise that the focus (especially at the early stages of strength development) is on technique rather than output. If they do not listen, I remind them of the song 'It ain't what you do, it's the way that you do it!' If they still don't listen, I sing it to them, and whilst my sister is an opera singer, I can't sing for toffee. My patients generally don't want a repeat performance so all I need to do to remind them is to threaten them with a song.

Advice

Throughout the exercises in this chapter – REMEMBER – focus on technique over effort. If you don't learn to do the exercises correctly from the start you will get into bad habits that will be hard to undo. If you do them correctly from the start, you should really move forwards and progress.

Getting some oomph back into your life

In life, you will frequently find you need some oomph to get things done properly. This may be the effort required to lift some shopping up a flight of stairs. It may be something less difficult, like opening a heavy shop door, or it could even be something as simple as standing up and pouring a cup of tea without spilling it everywhere. Some of the day-to-day challenges that you currently feel are beyond you might be manageable if you learn to harness breathing power. The power of the breath is what top sportsmen, dancers and even tradesmen use to maximise human performance to such extraordinary degrees.

Whilst you might think it rather odd to compare the training techniques of athletes to those of COPD patients, it is purely the fact that everyone else takes their breathing for granted that makes the two similar.

These groups of people are at polar ends of the fitness spectrum, but both have to work extra hard – the athletes to improve performance, the COPD patients to get what little air in that they can.

I have found that many of the breathing techniques that athletes use to maximise their performance also work very well for breathless patients. When you consider that the average Olympic heavyweight male rower could blow up 1000 party balloons in a race of just over five minutes, being able to take advantage of a small amount of that ability could provide extraordinary life-changing improvements in capacity for a person with COPD.

Earlier in this book, I explained how muscular action plays a key part in controlling the relative pressures in the chest and the abdominal cavities. If you remember, in Chapter 7 I detailed how the actions of the lower-body muscles needed to be equalised by the contraction of the muscles in the back and abdominals to maintain the alignment of the abdominal mass. By controlling the rate and force of exhalation (breathing out) you can help to ensure your body has a strong foundation to work from.

As a way of explaining this further, you just need to think about the effort a shot putter would put into throwing a 16 lb (7.25 kg) weight over 70 feet (21 metres). Think of how a shot putter seems to explode, with every muscle in their body from the tips of their toes to the tips of their fingers being essentially a single movement. If they are really putting every ounce of effort into the throw, they will inevitably yell as they throw. This yelling is not, as you might imagine, designed to attract attention, but is in fact sequenced to coincide with the expelling of the compressed air from the lungs as the body launches the shot away. Other sportsmen and women have their own way of coordinating their breath with a movement. You can't watch a professional tennis match without hearing a screech or shout as they serve. A karate exponent demonstrating a block break uses their full effort including a shout of 'Hoi'. Even with more gentle sports, breathing plays a key part in controlling human movement. Freestyle front crawl swimmers use a '3 stroke out and 1 stroke in' breath as standard, and even pistol shooters control their exhalation as they fire to ensure consistent and accurate results.

For some of the patients I see, getting out of a low chair requires the equivalent effort to a weight-lifter lifting a 200 kg barbell. For others, opening a door takes the same relative effort as a karate expert punching through a block of wood. It therefore makes sense that COPD patients can use similar breathing techniques to re-educate their bodies to coordinate their breath and the effort, at least until they have become stronger and can manage to take a more appropriate breath.

Simply put, the amount of force you need to use to carry out an activity needs to be equalised by the amount of force you put into your breathing. This is all relative to your abilities, so you will need to teach yourself how to take the appropriate volume of air into your lungs to help ensure you do not run out of breath during an activity. Whilst it takes practice to fine tune your relative physical and breathing effort, this will be quite simple as you will find out. The hard part will be to remember to prepare yourself to breathe before you do an activity that requires significant effort. Most patients forget to breathe, so preparing yourself mentally in advance is the biggest problem you will have to overcome.

When you think about how hard you need to breathe compared with the weight-lifter above, it seems obvious that a high level of effort requires more oomph and more controlled breathing, even before you think about it more deeply. Rather than explain in depth how you should breathe relative to the effort you are anticipating, I have put it all into Figure 9.1.

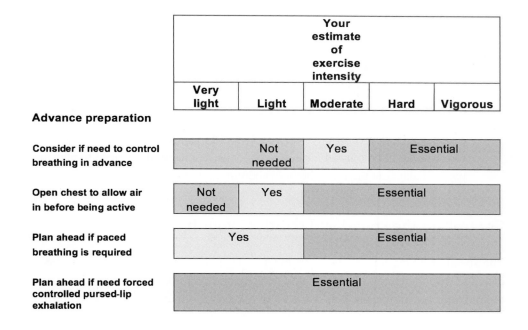

Figure 9.1: *Thinking ahead to breathe*

- Planning ahead if an exercise requires you to breathe in a certain way comes naturally to most of us when we are young and active. All you are doing is waking your mind up to do something that is completely natural to your body. Hopefully by this stage of the Brice Method, your brain is getting plenty of oxygen to make your thought processes clearer. A less fuzzy mind is one of the joys of natural relaxed breathing.

Inhalation during more vigorous exercise

Up to this stage I have trained you not to focus on inhalation. When you progress to this stage, you will need to start to consider if you have enough air in your lungs to execute an exercise, and if you are unable to prepare your posture to open your lungs fully, you may need to breathe in actively.

- **Inhalation during high levels of effort:** If the effort you are undertaking is very high relative to your strength or is quite complex relative to your physical abilities, you may need to take in extra air to give you enough air to keep some pressure in your lungs to work in tandem with the muscular effort of your limbs and torso. Doing so also enables you to maintain that effort for a significantly longer period of time.
- **Inhalation during gentle levels of effort:** At the other end of the spectrum, a very gentle degree of physical effort would mean that you would only have to take a small amount of air into your lungs, as they will not need to play any part in balancing the intra-thoracic/abdominal mass pressure.

Controlling the speed and depth of your breath

The speed at which you allow air to escape via pursed-lip exhalation will need to coincide with the length of activity you need to do. It is important that you do not try to hold your breath for any longer than 5 or 6 seconds without letting a little air out. If you do hold your breath, the pressure receptors in your lungs will start to signal a warning alarm to your brain, and make you feel particularly uncomfortable. If you hold for longer than 10 to 15 seconds under considerable effort, not only will your lungs be warning you of impending doom, but the level of oxygen in them and in your bloodstream will deplete enough to send even more emergency signals to your brain to drive you to breathe in an uncontrolled fashion similar to that of a severe bout of breathlessness (often known as an 'exacerbation').

The speed at which you release the air from your lungs plays an important part in retaining the air in your lungs long enough for oxygen to transfer into your bloodstream. As mentioned in the previous chapters, you should avoid letting all the air out too quickly. This is where you need to practise, slowly exhaling as you do the full range of motion. Sometimes the period of effort will exceed the time it takes you to count 'one thousand, two thousand, three thousand' (see page 62). Do not worry if this happens, simply let less air escape through your pursed lips to slow the flow and learn that you can also pace the exhalation in time with the exercise as easily as you can do it the other way around.

The use of your breath to aid performance plays a key part in almost every activity you can think of. The three main actions that this stage of the Brice Method will cover are pulling, pushing and lifting against a resistance. The means of resistance I will be recommending is to use a simple resistance tube.

Using resistance tubes

I find that resistance tubes are a great way to exercise without having to buy expensive equipment. An investment of approximately £10 on a resistance tube like the one shown in Figure 9.2, along with a simple door-jamb attachment that costs approximately £3, will give you the basic movements you might need, in a light and compact package.

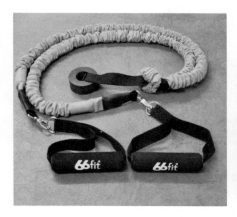
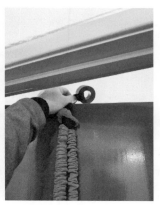

Figure 9.2: *Using resistance bands if needed*

Using a resistance band is relatively simple, but you do need to take care where you attach the band before you start exercising; the last thing you want is a door handle working its way loose from the stress of the band, and knocking you out as the band twangs towards you. The band should be fixed to a strong, solid mounting, such as a stair banister, or a wall-mounted safety bar. If you do not have stairs, you can make sure the resistance tube has a door-jamb attachment, so that you can fix it at any height between a closed door and the door-frame. Do ensure you push or pull against the direction of the door opening, as it will prevent the chance of the door opening under the pressure of effort, and also stop another person from opening the door as you are exercising, both of which could result in the band pinging towards you.

All three of the exercises described below can be executed seated or standing, depending upon your personal preference. If you decide to stand, do make sure that with each exercise you do not lock your knees straight. If you do this, you can put too much pressure on your lower back, so you are advised to stand with your knees slightly bent. This is called having soft knees, and this will ensure that all the force of working against the resistance bands is safely compensated for by your body.

Pulling against a resistance exercise

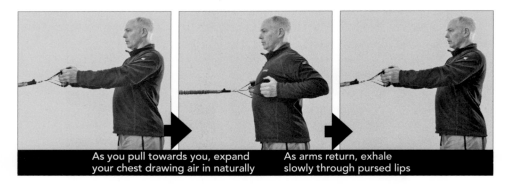

As you pull towards you, expand your chest drawing air in naturally

As arms return, exhale slowly through pursed lips

Figure 9.3: *Pulling against a resistance*

This first movement is a simple rowing movement, pulling a resistance towards you. This is almost exactly the same action as with the seated row exercise in Chapter 6 (page 73).

- Fix the exercise band to the door-jamb just below chest height.
- Stand or sit tall facing towards the door-jamb, with your hands straight out in front of you.
- Shuffle back away from the door until you have tension in the exercise band.
- Ensure your shoulders are drawn back and your head is looking straight ahead.
- Let air draw into your lungs naturally as you draw your elbows back.
- Remember, don't suck the air in.
- Exhale gently as you lower your arms back to the starting position.

Repeat the above sequence 10 times, exhaling for a count of 'one thousand, two thousand, three thousand' and inhaling for a count of 'one thousand'.

Fine-tuning the pulling resistance exercise

- Keep your knees slightly bent throughout the movement to protect your lower back.
- As you get slightly stronger and more confident with this you can move further away from the band fixing to increase the level of resistance.
- Initially, when there is only a small amount of resistance, you will not have to inhale or exhale actively, as your body does not need to over exert. You will soon notice that the resistance you have to pull against will need to be mirrored by the amount of effort you put into your breathing.

Note

The advice here goes somewhat against conventional practice for this exercise as it asks you to breathe in as you draw the elbows back. This is because it has been modified to suit COPD patients like you.

If you eventually start pulling significant weight in a gym setting, you may find that you need to adjust this technique, and exhale as you pull towards you. At this stage it is anticipated that you are not planning on entering any strongman or strongwomen contests; you are more likely to be simply wanting to do more mundane daily tasks around the home or in the garden.

Pushing against a resistance exercise

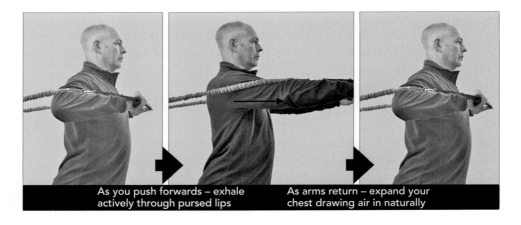

As you push forwards – exhale actively through pursed lips

As arms return – expand your chest drawing air in naturally

Figure 9.4: *Pushing against a resistance*

This exercise has many similarities to the wall press-up exercise completed in Chapter 6 (page 76).

- Hook the tube in the door fixing at about chest height and stand or sit tall facing away from the door.
- Take the slack out of the band by shuffling forwards away from the door.
- Keep your head up with your eyes looking parallel to the floor and hold your hands at shoulder height.
- Keep your knees slightly bent throughout the movement to protect your lower back.
- Exhale actively as you punch your hands forward away from you.
- Let air draw into your lungs naturally as you let your elbows draw back behind you towards the door.
- Remember, don't suck the air in.

Repeat the above sequence 10 times, exhaling for a count of 'one thousand, two thousand, three thousand' and inhaling for a count of 'one thousand'.

Fine-tuning the pushing against resistance exercise

- Stand with soft knees, especially if you have low back pain.
- Keep the door attachment, and your hands, at shoulder height. This will stop the band from twanging you around your ears.
- Remember that the further away from the door you move, the more resistance you will be expecting yourself to do as the resistance band stretches tighter.
- The amount of tension you have on the band will determine the degree of effort you will need to put into the exhaled breath. A low level of tension on the resistance band will need very little effort in exhalation, whereas a higher level of tension will mean you need to exhale more actively, through pursed lips.

Lifting against a resistance exercise

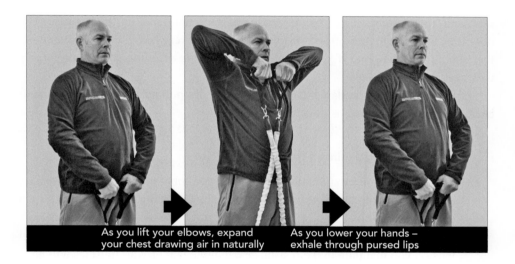

As you lift your elbows, expand your chest drawing air in naturally

As you lower your hands – exhale through pursed lips

Figure 9.5: *Lifting against a resistance*

The upright row (page 74) is an ideal exercise to help you learn the breathing pattern you should adopt when lifting something upwards towards your chest.

- Stand or sit tall with your shoulders drawn back and your head looking straight ahead.

- Stand on the resistance band with your hands lowered down in front of your hips.
- Keep your head up with your eyes looking parallel to the floor and hold your hands at shoulder height.
- Keep your knees slightly bent throughout the movement to protect your lower back.
- Let air draw into your lungs naturally as you lift your elbows drawn up high, with the thumbs pulling under your chin.
- Remember, don't suck the air in.
- Exhale gently as you lower your arms back to the starting position.

Repeat the above sequence 10 times, exhaling for a count of 'one thousand, two thousand, three thousand' and inhaling for a count of 'one thousand'.

Once more, the pacing of your breathing should be to count for 'one thousand, two thousand, three thousand' on the out phase and 'one thousand' on the in phase. The only time this should be adjusted is if you are lifting a very heavy weight, something that should only be done if you are physically capable of doing so, and preferably under correct supervision.

So, in summary, the fundamental is to inhale as you pull and lift upwards, as your chest should be expanding as the effort is executed.

Fine-tuning the lifting against a resistance exercise

- Tension the band by stretching and standing on more or less of it, making sure each arm is doing the same level of exercise by balancing out the length of each end of the band.
- As with the previous two exercises in this chapter, the greater the level of tension you maintain in the resistance band, the harder your muscles will have to work, and the greater the amount of effort you will subsequently have to put into the exhaled breath.

Note

Similar to the pulling-towards-you exercise before this, the advice for lifting against a resistance goes somewhat against conventional practice as you are asked to inhale as you lift. This is because it has been modified to suit COPD patients.

118

If you eventually start pulling significant weight in a gym setting, you may find that you need to adjust this technique and exhale as you lift. Once more it is anticipated that you are not planning on entering any strength competitions; you are more likely to be wanting to do simple jobs around the home.

Case study – Brian

Brian was 83 years old when I first met him. His breathing was shallow, fast and he got out of breath walking the 20 yards to the reception desk to meet me. Being an ex-paratrooper, Brian pushed himself as hard as he could before he started the programme, but even then, he was unable to take his little dog for a walk too far without having to stop and get his breath back.

On his first visit, Brian sat hunched in his chair, but quickly found that the postural exercises helped him. The penny dropped, and he soon mastered how to breathe and move, and then progressed to do more active exercises. After his rehabilitation ended, he joined the gym and being the competitive sort, started lifting weights with the big boys. We now have to stop him deadlifting a 100 kg bar, nearly twice his body weight! Whilst it is inspirational to see him feel so capable, we really do not recommend you attempt lifting such a weight yourself.

A further challenging movement – bending forwards

Bending forwards when you have COPD can be quite a challenge. If you think of the postural problems we have discussed to this point, with the diaphragm being compromised by the gut, it is logical that forward bending would have a very limiting effect on your breathing. To make matters worse, you may have developed some additional abdominal fat, perhaps as a result of being on frequent courses of steroids. There is no quick fix to reduce the size of the abdominal mass. Weight loss takes time and whilst it will eventually be a considerable help to ease the issue, we need to find alternative ways round the problem of forward bending and breathlessness. In reality, you have to bend forwards to do many everyday tasks, from tying your shoelaces to drying your feet, or cutting your toenails. It is true that most of you will have found alternative ways to avoid a good many of these activities, and you will probably already have taken to not wearing lace-up shoes, and using a chiropodist to cut your toenails. Figure 9.6 shows a simple exercise that needs to be practised quite specifically to address this issue. Just leaning forwards without thinking about your technique will definitely make you short of breath. Follow the technique and persevere with it and you are highly likely to get a little further forward, bit by bit. I can't, however, guarantee you will be cutting your own toenails again.

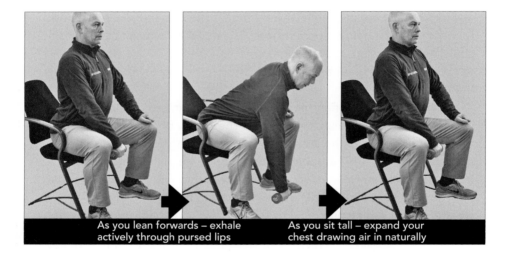

Figure 9.6: *Bending forwards*

Bending forwards seems like a simple exercise, until you can't do it.

- First you will need to sit down and perch forwards on an upright chair, sitting tall, drawing your shoulders back and trying to elongate the distance between your pubic bone and the bottom of your sternum. This will open your chest up and expand your lungs, giving you air to exhale later to help control the movement.
- You will then sit with your knees over your heels with your heels and knees wide apart.

- Your knees should preferably be wider than your shoulders and your hips.
- Once you are comfortable with this position you can then lean forward, ensuring you bend forward from the hip and not rounding your back. As you bend, immediately exhale as you lean forward. This exhalation will have the effect of slackening your diaphragm and allowing your abdominal mass to move up into the normal lung space.
- You will find that you will initially not want to hold yourself in this position for longer than 2 to 3 seconds, as your body may need a little time to acclimatise to the movement.
- As you lift your body back to the upright position allow the air to draw back into your lungs, aiding the process by returning to the upright, seated position with your shoulders drawn apart.

It may be that other muscle groups, such as your hamstrings, your lower back, middle back or shoulder joints, limit your ability to bend. These will also take time to get accustomed to the movement, a movement enabled by the control of the volume of air in your lungs.

Tracking your progress

In this chapter you should have learned how to prepare yourself to breathe at the correct level for the exercise you need to undertake. You should be able to pace your breathing with the movements and know when to exhale and when to inhale according to the movement you are doing.

Chapter 10

Skills for everyday life

◊ Conventional recovery positions for breathlessness
◊ The Brice Method recovery position
◊ Emotional breathing and COPD
◊ Panic breathing
◊ Hyperventilation syndrome
◊ Ssshh'ing technique to overcome hyperventilation
◊ Making natural, comfortable breathing a habit
◊ Being mindful
◊ Maintaining these habits for your lifetime
◊ Congratulations

Throughout the Brice Method, there is one theme that is consistent at each stage. This is that you should avoid getting out of breath to the point of discomfort. As you went through the simple postural exercises, the breathing exercises and sequencing the physical movements, you should have managed to feel calm and comfortable, rather than terribly short of breath. There will, however, be times when you do get breathless, either because you have overdone things, you are having an exacerbation, or you simply forgot to breathe as you have been trained to do. In this case, you will try to find a position of ease to recover.

Most COPD patients lean forward to catch their breath. This 'forward leaning posture' is the most commonly-taught recovery position, either if you are sitting or you are standing. It is true that the forward lean techniques can be of use, but their effectiveness is greatly reduced, if not nullified, if the exercises are not executed correctly. I have rarely seen anyone assume a completely effective lean forward posture, and feel that there is a need for the teaching points to be explained fully, or for another alternative to be taught. I will explain the relative benefits of each technique, as well as the fine-tuning teaching points that you will need to execute them well. I will also show the limitations of the techniques, and the alternative method I prefer to teach my patients using the Brice Method.

Conventional recovery positions for breathlessness

If you have already been shown recovery positions to help you get over a shortness of breath due to physical over-exertion, you are likely to have been shown one of the three forward leaning postures shown in Figure 10.1.

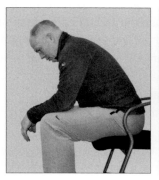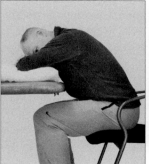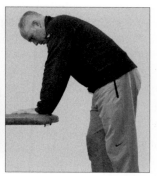

Figure 10.1: *Standard recovery positions: the seated forward lean posture, the supported head seated posture and the standing forward lean posture*

The seated forward lean posture

This is where you rest your elbows on your knees.

Potential benefits

- The idea is to lean forwards tilting the pelvis to allow the abdominal mass to topple forwards and give space for the diaphragm to work in.
- Resting the elbows on the knees is designed to take the weight of the arms off the neck muscles and partially lift the shoulder blades to open the rib cage a little more.

What many patients do wrong

- Most patients will bend forwards from the waist and not from the hips. If you tilt forwards from the waist the pelvis is fixed; as the pelvis does not rotate forwards the spine has to compensate by bending. This action forces the abdominal mass to push upwards into the diaphragm, preventing the diaphragm from working as it should. Bending forwards from the hips allows for a straighter spine enabling the pelvis and the abdominal mass to tilt forward as one, effectively reducing the upward pressure on the diaphragm.
- As shown in Figure 3.2 on page 41, a forward head position increases the stress on the muscles of the upper neck. Leaning forwards, close to 45 degrees from vertical, means that the strain on the trapezius and the four smaller 'capitis' muscle groups can exceed 22.5 kg – a physical stress that is hardly relaxing at any stretch of the imagination.
- As patients are unlikely to have been told to open their legs wide apart before they bend, they will usually keep their knees too close together. This is especially the case for women who have been taught decorum! Closed thighs not only limit the space for the abdominal mass to tip forwards, but increase the stress on the hamstring muscles, tilting the pelvis backwards, rather than forwards. Again, working totally against the object of the exercise.

The supported-head seated posture

This is where you lean forwards, arms on pillow on table, and head on arms.

Potential benefits

- If the exercise is executed properly, the abdominal mass is tilted forwards and can hang down between the legs, allowing the diaphragm space to contract and draw air into the lungs.
- By lifting the arms, the shoulder blades are drawn up, helping to expand the rib cage, and allowing the head to rest on the arms enables the neck muscles to relax temporarily and further reduces the stress to the body.

What many patients do wrong

- As with the exercise before, patients nearly always bend forwards, pivoting from the waist and not from the hips. Waist bending means the pelvis does not tip forwards and the abdominal mass is then pushed upwards towards the ribs, preventing the diaphragm from working.
- Again, as with the previous exercise, patients will rarely have been told to open their legs wide apart before they bend. Closing your thighs together prevents your abdominal mass from tipping forwards and stresses your hamstring muscles, tilting your pelvis backwards.

The standing forward lean posture

This is where you rest your hands on a table top or on your knees.

Potential benefits

- Similar to the seated lean, the standing lean forward aims to tilt the pelvis to allow the abdominal mass to topple forwards and give space for the diaphragm to work in.
- Resting the hands on a table or on the knees is designed to take the weight of the arms off the neck muscles and partially lift the shoulder blades to open the rib cage.

What many patients do wrong

- Most patients will bend forwards from the waist and not from the hips. If the back is not kept straight and the tilt done from the hips, the pelvis does not tip forwards and the abdominal mass pushes upwards, preventing the diaphragm from doing its job – completely counterproductive!
- As with the seated lean position, the forward head position increases the stress on the muscles of the upper neck, increasing the work the neck muscles have to do by as much as 350%.

These are relatively subtle differences, but because these exercises are rarely taught to take these issues into account, they can, and do, become bad habits in their own right.

The Brice Method recovery position

If you have already learned one of the leaning forward positions shown above, you may find this next exercise quite difficult to adopt at first; that is unless you have already truly mastered the postural exercises in this book. The reason it may be hard for you to unlearn the leaning techniques has been mentioned already: they may have become habitual to you. Habits such as these can be hard to break, so I suggest working on using this new technique at times when you are only slightly breathless from activity or stress. Once you have practised the technique, you can then progress to using it to overcome more physically or emotionally stressful situations. If you have worked through the book to this point, the technique should be simple for you.

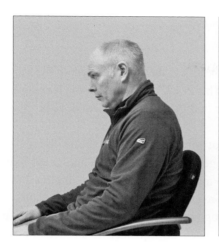 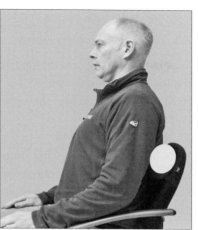

Figure 10.2: *The Brice Method recovery positon: Slumping (left) can cause restriction and tension in the chest, whereas sitting tall with a support under the shoulder blades (right) can open up the chest.*

- Sit down on a firm, high-backed chair, with your bottom right back into the seat, or stand against a wall.
- Place a rolled-up towel or back support pad, below and between your shoulder blades. The rolled-up towel or pad should be big enough for you to feel it push against your ribs as you lean backwards, but not so big that you are being pushed so that you lean forwards excessively.
- Draw your shoulder blades backwards and downwards, whilst simultaneously drawing the nape of your neck backwards. The towel or back support will act as a pivot point, allowing your ribs to open up like a fan, and will artificially expand your chest in the process.
- As you draw your shoulders backwards and downwards, you may find that your hands will need to fall by your hips or slide back on the arms of your chair. Work with this by putting your hands on your hips if your chair has no arm rests, or drawing your elbows back if your chair has them. If you are standing you can place your hands on your hips or behind your lower back.
- Once you are able to sit or stand in this position comfortably, you should then practise the usual paced breathing that you have used throughout the book. This is to count 'one thousand, two thousand, three thousand' as you breathe

out, and 'one thousand' as you breathe in.

How this recovery position works

- With the head balanced on top of the spine, the stress placed on the muscles in the back of the neck is only 5 kg. This is 17.5 kg less than the leaning forward head positions, enabling the upper body to be more relaxed, rather than tight and stressed.
- The back support helps act as a pivot point on the spine to allow the ribs to open up, which in turn draws the rib cage up and outwards. This means that there is extra space for the diaphragm to move downwards on inhalation. Inhalation will feel relatively easy, and be more comfortable.
- The upright stance means that the top two ribs are already elevated. This means that the accessory muscles of the neck do not need to be activated during inhalation, again reducing the level of muscular tension and stress.
- The shoulder blades are both drawn back, down and inwards towards the middle of the back, placing additional leverage on the posterior part of the rib cage, further flaring and elevating the ribs.
- The weight of the arms is behind the centre of gravity, helping counterbalance the whole shoulder girdle against the anterior rib cage and pectoral muscles.
- The paced breathing technique of 'three thousand' and 'one thousand' helps slow down the respiration rate to approximately 15 breaths per minute, allowing effective transfer of oxygen in the lungs and controlling the release of carbon dioxide.
- Most of the actions described above directly increase the volume of the lungs, and help reduce air pressure in the lungs relative to the external environment. This one simple reaction will not only reduce the amount of effort and energy required to inhale, but will also help the patient to relax and breathe more naturally.

Emotional breathing and COPD

It will be of little surprise to any person with severe breathlessness, be it related to COPD or not, that emotional upsets can set off an exacerbation.

Many of the causal factors that lead to severe breathlessness are found in patients who are relatively inactive, who have long-term medical complaints or who find themselves in a lot of pain. Many of my patients have stress from work or unemployment, and others are high achievers with perfectionist tendencies. Some of my patients find that boredom, phobias or anxiety are enough to set off a bad turn. Whilst there are many emotional triggers that can induce a bout of breathlessness, the three issues that my COPD patients consistently talk to me about are: fear, frustration and embarrassment.

- **Fear:** I can think of no emotion that is more powerful and more frightening than not being able to breathe. The human body can survive without water for many hours, and without food for days, but it can only last a couple of minutes without breathing. The body's emergency response mechanism kicks in quite quickly.
- **Frustration:** The anger at not being able to do what would have appeared to be a simple task a few years before, is another emotion that patients say makes them feel really frustrated. It is another deep emotion that can drive the physical manifestation of discomfort when they are breathless.
- **Embarrassment:** For some it can be mortifying to start having an exacerbation in public. This emotion can fan the flames of breathlessness, especially in an area where people are watching or crowding round to help you by asking you questions.

The answer to coping with the emotional issues that accompany breathing problems is to be able to recognise the issues and then learn how to manage your response to them. Your response might be to think in advance of doing any activity that you know will put physical strain on your body and begin to increase your breathing depth relative to the exercise you are about to do rather than wait to get breathless. It might be that you anticipate emotional cues that you know will elicit a physical response of breathlessness, and either avoid the situation or try to mitigate the effect of the stressor by adopting a more upright and powerful body position prior to the stress occurring. If you have already become breathless it might mean that you need to use the recovery position to reduce the physical stress on your body, and focus on paced breathing to slow your breathing down to comfortable levels quickly and easily.

Panic breathing

For those of us that have never had an exacerbation, or been unable to breathe due to over-exertion, the closest thing you are likely to have experienced is having your head dunked in water without warning. This feeling of fear and dread is primal, so it is little wonder that the body tells you to avoid anything that will cause a repeat episode at all costs. Sheer panic is the emotional response that we experience when we can't get enough air in, and by panicking, the body automatically and uncontrollably increases the rate of breathing, This makes our breath shallower, further reducing the amount of air reaching the depths of our lungs.

More often than not, panic will drastically affect breathing rate and depth detrimentally. The increase in breathing rate and depth that panic induces seems to have little or no impact on the amount of oxygen that reaches the bloodstream. This is partly due to the fact that a fast breath means any air that goes into the lungs has very little time in the alveoli to enable it to be absorbed into the bloodstream, and partly due to the fact that quick breaths tend to be more shallow, so the air does not actually go as deep into the lung as it otherwise would. Combine this with the fact that in a panic situation, most people will tend to hunch forwards to protect themselves (as if in the foetal position), reducing the capacity of the lungs and further reducing the effectiveness of the breath. As this effect continues to reduce the amount of oxygen in the bloodstream, the breathing rate is gradually sped up, and a spiralling feedback loop of ever-reducing oxygen levels only stops when the person is able to regain control of their breathing, or they get taken to accident and emergency under blue lights.

By their very nature, panic attacks happen with little or no warning, so it is unlikely that you will be able to plan ahead or rationalise the issues that have caused the problem. The immediate threat that your body feels it is under when its supply of oxygen is restricted can be very severe. From my experience, if you start to use the Brice Method recovery position, along with the paced breathing technique, you should be able to learn how to overcome panic breathing relatively easily. If you successfully manage to overcome panic-induced breathlessness a few times, it is likely that you will soon become less frightened of it happening and gain confidence that you can overcome it without having to require medical support. Having this confidence acts to reassure you that whilst at the time the panic is real, the consequences are far less problematic than your body's warning signals are telling you.

Hyperventilation syndrome

Having consistent, acute bouts of over-breathing is known clinically as 'hyperventilation syndrome'. This is recognised as a condition that is initiated by over-breathing, and is where too much carbon dioxide is being exhaled from the lungs. Just as the body wants to balance the blood oxygen levels, it also needs to maintain the correct amount of carbon dioxide in the bloodstream to balance the blood pH to 7.365. The body responds to imbalances in blood pH and relatively low levels of carbon dioxide not as you would think, by slowing down the breath, but by speeding the rate of breathing up!

Controlled, paced, deep nasal breathing normally combats hyperventilation. Here you breathe in through your nose for a count of 4, hold your breath momentarily and then let the air out for a count of 4. Whilst I have argued the case against nasal breathing elsewhere in this book, hyperventilation is an instance where you can and should use the technique, especially if you feel yourself to be very panicky or distressed. Slowing your breathing rate down to this pace is a little stressful, but it does bring your respiration rate down to between 10 and 12 breaths per minute, which is enough time to allow carbon dioxide levels to rebalance themselves.

Whilst controlled nasal breathing can work well when you are really panicking and breathless, I have found that I rarely need to use these methods with my patients, as I do not work them to the point where they get truly out of breath. In fact, I have found the most effective way of overcoming hyperventilation is to calm your breathing down by using what I call the 'ssshh'ing technique' (see Figure 10.3).

Ssshh'ing technique to overcome hyperventilation

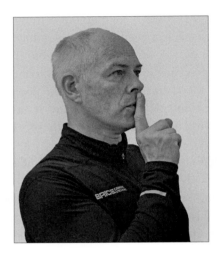

Figure 10.3: *Ssshh'ing exercise*

- You will need once again to adopt the upright body position to help de-stress your whole body system.
- You will need to use the paced (count 'one thousand, two thousand, three thousand' out, 'one thousand' in) breathing method to slow down your breathing rate to approximately 15 breaths a minute.
- Put one finger in front of your pursed lips, as if you are telling yourself to ssshh....
- You then actively hiss 'ssshh' as you count your 'three thousand' exhalation. This works really well to increase the pressure of all the gases in your lungs, and helps you to be actively thinkng that you are quietening your breathing down.
- You should continue to do this upright posture, ssshh, paced breathing technique unitl your breathing has settled down.

It may seem odd, that such a simple technique as this should work so effectively on what is a highly charged and extremely emotional situation. It appears that the ssshh'ing acts to help soothe you, in exactly the same way that a deep sigh makes you feel relaxed.

Making natural, comfortable breathing a habit!

Now that you have got to this stage in the Brice Method, you should be armed with the tools to continue to develop your own breathing coping strategies for whatever you want to do in your day-to-day life. You will obviously be restricted to the remaining capacity of your lungs, and the other bodily limitations you have. I work on a daily basis with a great many patients who thought they were on their last legs but who have not only stopped the decline of their physical abilities, but have also managed to regain considerable levels of fitness.

Being mindful

To maintain your progress, you will have to continue to be mindful of your body and of how much your breathing will limit you if you forget to breathe! You should now know how you can amend your posture, and avoid slumping back into your old ways. You should remember that you have to consider the breathing methods you need to use in advance of any activity you do. You will also need to focus on pacing your breath if you have to be active for a protracted length of time, and that you will have to synchronise your breath with the movements you do.

Failure to be mindful of any of these factors is likely to end up with you feeling dissatisfied with your breathing.

Maintaining these new habits for your lifetime

What you can do to help you maintain your improved breathing techniques is remember the listening exercise you did right at the beginning of the programme and at each stage of the Brice Method.
1.   Notice where your head is in relation to your body.
2.   Notice how you are holding your shoulders.

3. Think about the pace and speed of your breathing.
4. Recognise how deep the breath is going into your lungs.
5. Think about how satisfying each breath is.

When you can feel the difference, this will help you visualise what you are doing and make a mental map of your breathing. Visualising your body alignment and breathing pattern will help you to remember what you should do if you get breathless in the future and gives you a coping strategy that works for you. Even if you have been fixed in a slumped position due to inactivity caused by illness, injury or simple laziness for years, you can usually improve your posture by being self-aware of how much better your breathing is when you do not slump, and by doing the exercises that you feel work best for you several times a day.

Congratulations

You have now completed the final active part of the Brice Method. There are three addenda to this book that are designed to help provide additional support to patients with COPD who will need motivation and information to continue to benefit from the Brice Method.

- **Addendum 1** shows the results and feedback from my patients who have undertaken the Brice Method, gathered during the 12 months before completing this book.
- **Addendum 2** gives information about suitable equipment that can be used to help you get the most out of your exercises, plus details of how you can get more personalised assistance if you want to take the Brice Method further.
- **Addendum 3** is purely a list of the diagrams in the book. This quick reference guide might assist you if you want to look back at any of the images, especially if you are a person who finds visual cues and feedback useful.

I then only have left to say, very best wishes for continuing improvements in your breathing and fitness.

Addendum 1

Results and patient feedback

◊   **Results part A – Patient oxygen saturation levels**
◊   **Results part B – Patient self-reported quality of breath**
◊   **Results part C – Patient feedback**

Over the last few years of working within the NHS, I have found that other health professionals have become aware of, and more interested in, the techniques I use. This is mainly due to the positive feedback that I have received from some of the more demanding patients. These are the patients who might normally have not taken up, let alone benefited from, pulmonary rehabilitation. Despite this, some practitioners have remained dismissive of the techniques I use, so I decided to gather information specifically about the benefit patients have felt they gained just from the first introductory session.

Over the last year I have collected all the comments and scoring for the self-reported quality of breath test (SRQoB). This mirrors the scores of the first and second Landmark self-tests that you should have completed in this book. This means you can compare your scores and your assessment of any changes that you have made to 207 other COPD patients.

I use these results as a strong argument as to why the Brice Method could be a first-stage intervention for COPD, giving patients an opportunity to make lifestyle changes before they are given lifelong medication, or potentially delaying patients' need to use these drugs in the first place. Adopting the Brice Method at an early stage might even help save considerable sums of money for the NHS in the UK, as well as reduce the ongoing treatment caused by the potential harm of any side effects these drugs may have.

There are three parts to the patient evaluations included in this addendum:
- The first part gives the statistical results, showing the change from the start to the end of the introductory session, for the patients' blood oxygen saturation levels.
- The second part shows the mean results of the change in the self-reported quality of breath score between the start and the end of the introductory session.
- The third part shows the patient feedback as to how they felt having completed the first introductory session.

Results

Patient oxygen saturation levels

I measured 240 patients' oxygen saturation levels before the start and at the end of their first session. Oxygen saturation is a measure of how much oxygen the blood is carrying as a percentage of the maximum it can carry. Needless to say, COPD limits the capacity of the lungs to get oxygen into the bloodstream, so anything we can do for patients to increase this score in the long term is very useful.

Table A1.1: *COPD patient oxygen saturation levels*

Mean pre SPo2	Mean post SPo2	Mean variance %	Number of patients recorded
94.5%	97.6%	3.3%	240

By themselves these oxygen saturation scores are not the most effective means of evaluating how much a patient has benefited from using the first stages of the Brice Method. This said, I have found that being able to show an average increase of 3.1 out of 10 in such a short space of time works extremely well to motivate patients who might have been rather sceptical at the start of their first session. Many patients are genuinely surprised that they can do something themselves to increase the levels of oxygen in their bloodstream. I can only guess that they had previously thought that their lungs were damaged to the point of being useless, and they had no way of redressing the situation, especially when most had been told their lungs are irreparably damaged when they were first diagnosed as having COPD.

I remind patients that their lungs will not heal or recover from the damage that has been done to them; all I am doing is teaching them to use the remaining healthy part of their lungs as well as possible. In most instances this is more than enough for daily living activities, and in some cases it is much more.

Patient self-reported quality of breath scores

If you have already completed the exercises in this book you will have recorded your own self-reported quality of breath in the Landmark self-tests. These are a visual analogue scale and give a scoring from 1 to 10. On this scale, a score of 1 is poor, and a score of 10 is fantastic.

Table A1.2: *Self-reported quality of breath score evaluation (SRQoB)*

Mean pre-SRQoB	Mean post-SRQoB	Mean SRQoB variance	SRQoB % improvement	n=
4.77	7.83	3.08	64.5%	302

These mean scores are quite incredible. For patients to get a 64.5% improvement within the first introductory session not only makes them realise that they need to do the exercises regularly, but that they can actually do something other than take medication to help themselves breathe better! Scientifically the results might be seen as insignificant or that they are susceptible to influence from the practitioner, but for the patients themselves, these scores can be a highly beneficial eye opener.

Out of the 302 patients, only one person reported that their breathing felt worse after doing the exercises. Six patients said they felt no change but a staggering 295 said they felt that their breathing had improved. The average score at the start of the session, after they had been given time to settle down and get over their journey in to my clinic, was 4.77 out of 10. At the end of the session the average score was 7.83 out of 10. The individual scores that make up these averages are shown in Table A1.3.

Table A1.3: *Change in SRQoB score*

Change in SRQoB score	Number of patients	% of Total
-1	1	0%
0	6	2%
1	25	8%
2	72	24%
3	98	32%
4	54	18%
5	25	8%
6	10	3%
7	10	3%
8	0	0%
9	0	0%
10	1	0%

As you can imagine, I am always excited when patients have felt dramatic improvements, and this is why I am so committed to promoting the Brice Method. If this were a drug, it could be one of the most effective medications for people suffering from COPD.

Hopefully, your own Landmark test scores throughout this book have shown similar results.

Patient feedback

Whilst statistical results can show quantitative variations, I wanted to gather more qualitative feedback from patients. After asking them how they would rate their breathing on a score of 1 to 10, I then asked them, 'How would you describe how your breathing feels now?'

Looking at the word frequency from all of the feedback quotes, this demonstrates most clearly what patients felt. The chart on the next page shows the number of times patients mentioned a particular word or set of words to describe how their breathing was after completing the first session with me.

Table A1.4: *COPD patients' experience of the introductory session of the Brice Method*

It feels better	56
Breathe deeper	38
More relaxed	30
It is easier	25
Feel difference	24
Amazing	21
Lungs more open	16
Expands chest	11
More comfortable	10
Unbelievable	9
More aware	7
Feels very good	7
Not short of breath	6
Not struggling	6
Feel it all over	6
Brilliant	6

Below I have included some of the more interesting quotes that my patients have given. This will give you some idea of the varied responses I have had:

- 'I don't feel as out of breath. I feel more relaxed and I am not thinking about it as much.'
- 'I was sceptical that this would help but I can feel my chest more able to take air in.'
- 'It feels more controlled. Not as if I am gasping as much. It is easier and feels nice and natural.'
- 'I can feel the breath throughout my lungs, I feel less congested and my breathing feels much easier which gives me confidence.'
- 'I feel 100% better than when I walked in. I feel full of air now.'
- 'I thought I was breathing ok until I was shown how to breathe. I can now feel my lungs expanding.'

- 'I feel that I can breathe properly. You wouldn't believe this would help you breathe so well.'
- 'It is pretty amazing. I don't have my oxygen on and I feel relaxed. It is silly. I feel like I am taking a lungful of air now.'
- 'I usually feel phlegm rattling in my neck, now I don't feel it.'
- 'It feels marvellous. I don't feel like I am fighting for my breath.'
- 'It feels better. I don't know why my doctor has never told me this.'
- 'It sounds weird but I feel more open and I am not as panty. It feels I have more space and the brick wall I usually have is not there.'
- 'Breathing seems easier almost immediately. There is a noticeable difference.'
- 'This is ridiculous. I couldn't walk in here without being breathless, I just walked up the road and back and I am not out of breath at all.'

If you are interested in reading all of the feedback quotes to get more insight into exactly how all the patients felt, you can contact me through my website www.paulbrice.net, and I will forward them to you.

I hope that you will take inspiration from these comments from my COPD patients and realise you are in very good company as you undertake the Brice Method.

Addendum 2

Equipment and further advice

I have included this section as I am aware that many of my patients have struggled to know what equipment to use when they have had to do the exercises at home rather than in the gym environment. It goes through the options that you can choose to take, with some of the pros and cons of each, be it suitability, effectiveness or cost.

Equipment you might need to start off

Initially in the Brice Method, the only equipment you need is an upright chair and a method of supporting your rib cage just below your shoulder blades. This is what you will have carried out in Exercise 1 in Chapter 4 (page 48). To execute this exercise correctly you need to choose a back support that gives your body adequate assistance. You may find that your needs change as your body adapts to the exercise, so I am adding a full description of the benefits of the various back supports you can use, as well as ready-made options you can purchase.

Choosing the best back support for you

To start off with no cost, roll up a towel

Initially, I recommend my patients use a rolled-up towel to support their back (see Figure A2.1). Not only are they easy to find, they also provide a gentle support that pushes against three or four ribs at a time. They are generally comfortable to use, and once you have learned how to roll them up so that they stay in place and suit your needs, they can be sewn up or tied to the chair so that they don't unfurl all the time.

Get a medium-sized towel and fold it in half lengthways. Then roll it up to about half way along and drape it over the back of your upright chair with the roll facing to the chair. You will have to guestimate how far down the back of the chair the belly of the roll sits, so that it will be located under and between your shoulder blades. Gravity and friction should hold the rolled-up towel in place long enough for you to sit down and position yourself correctly.

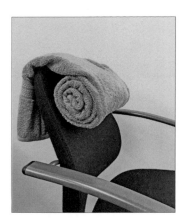

Figure A2.1: *Rolled towel as back support*

Ready-made alternative: lumbar roll

If you get on well with the towel, but find it fiddly trussing it up or tying it in place, you can buy bespoke back supports that do a better job and stay in place. They are often called lumbar supports, and whilst you will need to use them differently from what they were designed for, they are made of a spongy roll, with a soft covering and an elasticated strap that is adjustable to fit your chair. These are soft and gentle on your back whilst providing support over three or four ribs at a time.

Both of these supports provide quite a general level of support across the full width of the ribs. They tend to be comfortable but do not really push the body to the same degree as the more direct support options that I will explain next (see Figure A2.2).

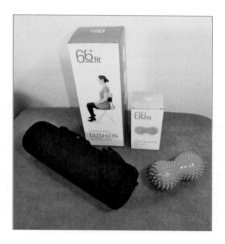

Figure A.2.2: *A lumbar roll (left) and a spikey peanut roll (right)*

Ready-made alternative: spikey peanut

The spikey peanut is designed specifically to stimulate and make you aware of your body. The peanut shape means it fits perfectly against the ribs whilst ensuring no pressure is placed on the spine itself. The little spikes are designed to apply pressure to the muscles of the back, and more specifically to help release 'trigger points' in the muscles to help them relax, much in the same way a massage therapist would do.

The home-made alternative to the spikey peanut

If you do not feel that you get much support from the towel or spongy roll, you might prefer the more direct approach using something a little firmer. Get two tennis balls and an old sock. Put one of the balls into the sock and tie the sock just above the tennis ball to keep it in place. Repeat this with the second tennis ball and you will have a peanut shaped support you can place in your back. You will need to ensure the balls are horizontal to the floor, pushed against the back of the chair below and in between your ribs. Do not position the balls so that they directly push on your spine. Whilst it is unlikely to damage your spine, the individual vertebrae do not like direct pressure placed upon them; they will soon tell you not to do it, as it will be uncomfortable.

Once you have tried the different options of back support you will also be able to fine-tune the placing of the supports to best suit your body. Not only is everyone different, but also as you get more and more used to using the support over time, your body may eventually change shape, and you may find that you need to alter the position of the support to obtain the most benefit.

In my clinic, I tend to use a spikey peanut with my patients as a way of getting very specific support to the rib cage, as shown in Figure 4.3, earlier in the book (page 53).

Resistance equipment

For the arm exercises to develop strength in Chapter 9, I have suggested the use of an exercise band with a door attachment. These can be purchased either as exercise bands, bungee cords or resistance bands. They are relatively inexpensive – £20 will get you a band and a door anchor delivered to you. You will only need a door anchor if you do not have a strong banister or handrail to wrap the resistance band around.

Alternatively, you can use a light dumbbell; if you are light, a 2 kg dumbbell will suffice. If you are heavier and quite strong you can go up to 5 kg without too much difficulty. Examples of these are shown in Figure A2.3.

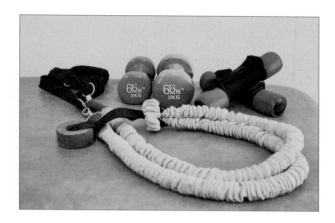

Figure A2.3: *Resistance band with door anchor attached to it (front left) with dumbbells (to the rear)*

Further advice and support

This book is designed as a self-help guide. For some patients with COPD this guide will be self-explanatory and the various exercises will feel very simple to follow. If, however, you feel that you would benefit from additional support, then you can find more details about personalised support packages from my website: www.paulbrice.net

Daily homework tracking sheets

Copies of the daily tracking sheet may be of use, so here is a full five weeks' worth for photocopying. You can also download them from my website.

You can track your daily activity on the tables so that you ensure you repeat the homework exercises four times a day. Mark X in the relevant box for every time you do one group of the exercise routines.

Week 1	Monday	Tuesday	Wednesday	Thursday	Friday	Saturday	Sunday
Early morning							
Mid morning							
Afternoon							
Evening							

Week 2	Monday	Tuesday	Wednesday	Thursday	Friday	Saturday	Sunday
Early morning							
Mid morning							
Afternoon							
Evening							

© Paul Brice, 2018

Week 3	Monday	Tuesday	Wednesday	Thursday	Friday	Saturday	Sunday
Early morning							
Mid morning							
Afternoon							
Evening							

Week 4	Monday	Tuesday	Wednesday	Thursday	Friday	Saturday	Sunday
Early morning							
Mid morning							
Afternoon							
Evening							

Week 5	Monday	Tuesday	Wednesday	Thursday	Friday	Saturday	Sunday
Early morning							
Mid morning							
Afternoon							
Evening							

Addendum 3

List of figures

Index

Note: bold page numbers show the page where full information on each Landmark can be found.

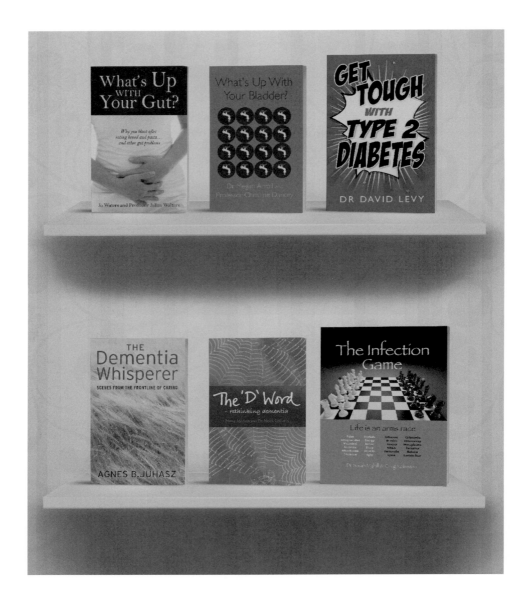